I0448918

Clear Mind, Confident Self

A Woman's Guide to Menopausal Mental Wellness

by
Well-Being Publishing

To You,

Thank you!

Table of Contents

Introduction:
Embracing the Journey

Welcome to the gateway of a profound shift, a time in life where transformation is not just about the body, but equally the mind. As you stand at the threshold of menopause, you're embarking on a journey that's as challenging as it is empowering. Think of this as an exploration, where each step is an opportunity for growth and deeper understanding of your mental milieu. You're not alone on this path. Many have walked it before, and through these pages, you'll glean insights, strategies, and heartfelt advice to navigate the mental and emotional waves that come with the menopausal transition. We'll extend beyond mere coping mechanisms, striving for thriving—a mental state blossomed from informed choices and positive actions. Embrace this guide as a beacon, illuminating the twists and turns with grace and knowledge, ensuring you emerge resilient, rejuvenated, and ready for the wonders that await in post-menopause.

Understanding Menopause

Having just embraced the idea of the menopausal journey, it's time to dive into what menopause really entails, unraveling it layer by layer. At its core, menopause is not just a biological transition; it represents a pivotal moment in a woman's life where experiences can vary as widely as the individuals themselves. Hormones are shifting, and yes, it can feel like a roller coaster—complete with ups, downs, and the occasional loop-the-loop. It's a time that can be tangled up in myths and misconceptions, from aging fears to misconceptions about its impact on our vitality and mental sharpness. This chapter isn't about feeding into those myths. It's about setting the record straight, examining the

1

facts, and understanding our bodies—all to equip us with the power to navigate this change with confidence. Let's begin this chapter with the assurance that menopause, while complex, isn't a cloud without a silver lining. It's an opportunity to understand ourselves on a deeper level, to harness the wisdom of our bodies, and to debunk the tales that have long shadowed the truth of this natural life stage.

The Biological Transition

As we wave goodbye to the reproductive chapter of our lives, the biological transition known as menopause becomes our new reality. It's a natural phase, one defined by the end of menstrual cycles, but here's what's fascinating: it's not an off-switch but rather a gradual dimming that our bodies control through a complex symphony of hormonal fluctuations. Picture this—the ovaries are the grand conductors, their batons slowing, altering the rhythm of estrogen and progesterone. This shift can trigger a cascade of physical and emotional changes. And while each woman's experience is uniquely her own, common threads weave through the tapestry of this transition. Understanding what's happening internally empowers us to navigate the changes with grace and wisdom instead of fear. So let's dive into this chapter with curiosity and a willingness to learn, because grasping the biological transition is our first step in mastering this new stage of life.

Hormonal Changes and Their Psychological Impact

The journey of menopause isn't just about the physical manifestations—it's a mental marathon too. As we turn the page from the biological underpinnings of menopause, it's crucial to examine the profound psychological effects imbued by hormonal fluctuations. Understanding these changes can empower you to navigate this transition with grace and strength.

Hormones like estrogen and progesterone don't just govern the menstrual cycle; they're pivotal in regulating brain chemistry. During menopause, as the levels of these hormones decline, you might find that you're not just losing your periods, but also, at times, feeling like you're losing your mind!

One moment you're on top of the world, the next, you could be plummeted into the depths of irritability or sadness without a visible cause. These mood swings aren't a sign of weakness; they're a natural response to the chemical changes happening within your body. Recognizing this can be affirming and can reduce the self-blame or confusion you may be experiencing.

Anxiety is another frequent flyer in the menopausal skies. You might find yourself worrying excessively about things that previously felt manageable. Remember, this isn't you overreacting; it's your body trying to adapt to a new hormonal balance. Awareness of this fact can be the first step toward seeking comfort and solutions.

Sleep disturbances are often closely linked to hormonal upheaval, hence the night sweats and insomnia. Poor sleep can affect your mood, cognitive function, and overall mental health. While we won't dive into sleep solution specifics here, understanding that hormonal changes are often the root cause can pave the way for seeking appropriate remedies.

Self-image can also take a hit during menopause. Fluctuating weight, changes in skin condition, and body shape can affect how you perceive yourself, sparking feelings of inadequacy or a lack of confidence. It's vital to remind yourself that these changes are natural and part of a process that every menopausal woman experiences.

Depression, or a significant depressive mood, catches some women off guard. If you find yourself feeling persistently sad or hopeless, it's not just "in your head." Hormonal shifts can be potent influencers on your emotional state, and acknowledging this can be the bridge toward professional support and healing.

Concentration and memory can sometimes feel like they're betraying you. If you walk into a room and forget why, or struggle to focus like you used to, it's not necessarily age catching up with you. It could be your hormones, playing with your cognitive functions like a puppeteer with strings.

Sexual desire can wax and wane unpredictably, leaving you feeling disconnected from your own sensuality or from your partner. It's not a lack of love or attraction; it's often the hormonal roller coaster rerouting your libido. Patience and open communication become key assets during this time.

You might also notice increased sensitivity to stress or a feeling of being overwhelmed by tasks that you once handled with ease. This can trigger a stress response that's disproportionate to the challenge at hand. Knowing that this heightened stress response is tied to hormonal fluctuations can help you seek stress management strategies that work for you.

During this time, nihilistic thoughts may creep in: "Is this all there is?" or "What's the point?" This existential unease isn't uncommon, and while partly philosophical, it's also tied to the hormonal-induced shifts in brain chemistry. Grounding yourself in purposeful activities can reignite a sense of meaning and direction.

With this cavalcade of psychological shifts, you might feel like you're standing on shifting sands. Nonetheless, grasping the hormonal etiology behind these feelings can be a powerful tool in regaining steadiness. It's by understanding the why that we can better strategize the how when it comes to coping mechanisms and interventions.

So, as we navigate through this often bumpy ride, let's remember that empowerment comes through knowledge. While hormones play their symphony—and at times it might feel more like a cacophony—by understanding their effects on our mental well-being, we can tune our self-care practices to maintain harmony in our lives.

Lastly, while it's important to normalize these experiences, never normalize suffering. If you feel the psychological impact of hormonal changes is too much to bear, it's imperative to reach out for professional help. This isn't a time for stoic solitude, but rather for community, understanding, and support.

Remember, the wrinkles in our brains are just as important as those on our skin. We might not be able to smooth out the former, but we certainly can ensure they don't define the landscape of our mental health. With this understanding, we can embrace the changes, responsive to our needs, armed with strategies, and supported by a community that understands our journey.

Myths and Facts about Menopause

When it comes to menopause, there's an abundance of myths and misconceptions floating around that can muddle our understanding of this significant life transition. It's time to demystify some of these fallacies and shine a light on the truths that will empower you as you embark on this journey.

First off, there's the prevailing myth that menopause marks the beginning of a decline, being synonymous with old age. Let's set the record straight: menopause is not a marker for becoming 'old'. Rather, it's a natural biological process that occurs as a part of maturing—an experience that every woman goes through. The transition into menopause, also known as perimenopause, can start as early as your 40s, and it's simply a shift into a new phase of life.

Another common myth is the idea that menopause leads to an inevitable gain in weight. While hormonal changes can indeed affect your metabolism and body composition, it's not a foregone conclusion that weight gain is unavoidable. With mindful eating and regular physical activity—the same advice given at any stage of life—maintaining a healthy weight is entirely possible.

Some believe that a plummet in sexual desire is guaranteed during menopause. Here's the fact: while hormonal changes can sometimes affect libido, it doesn't spell the end of your sex life. Many women find that freedom from concerns about pregnancy and an increase in self-confidence can actually lead to a revitalized interest in sex.

Let's address the idea that mood swings during menopause are just 'all in your head'. In truth, the hormonal changes can have a very real impact on your emotions. However, that doesn't mean you're destined for emotional turmoil. There are plenty of strategies and treatments available that can help you manage mood swings effectively.

There's also the misconception that hormone replacement therapy (HRT) is dangerous for all women. It's essential to understand that HRT, like any medical treatment, has its risks and benefits, which can vary greatly from person to person. It's not a one-size-fits-all approach, and with medical guidance, many women find HRT to be a helpful part of their menopause strategy.

Another myth making the rounds is that menopause results in the loss of cognitive function. While some may experience issues with concentration or memory during menopause, these symptoms are typically temporary. Cognitive health can be maintained through various lifestyle factors such as diet, exercise, and mental activities.

Moving on, there's the myth that all women experience severe menopausal symptoms. In reality, every woman's experience is different. Some may have significant symptoms while others barely notice the transition. Understanding this can help moderate expectations and alleviate unnecessary anxiety about the process.

One of the less talked about myths is that life becomes less fulfilling after menopause. Quite the contrary—many women report feeling more liberated and energized without the inconvenience of periods and the unpredictability of PMS. It's a time that can be marked by personal growth and new ventures.

Also, debunking the myth that menopause is an illness that needs to be 'cured' is crucial. Menopause is a natural part of life, not a medical condition. While some symptoms may require management, this period doesn't inherently necessitate medical intervention. It's an opportunity to recalibrate your lifestyle and focus on wellness.

There's also a false belief that only women experience menopause. Well, while the term 'menopause' is specific to women, it should be noted that men go through a comparable (though not identical) transition known as andropause. Acknowledging this underscores that transitions are a part of life for everyone.

Lastly, there's the myth that menopause is the same for every woman. The truth couldn't be further from this. Ethnicity, health history, lifestyle, and even your attitude toward menopause can influence your experience. It's highly personalized and that's why the journey is unique for each individual.

In conclusion, sifting through the myths to uncover the truths about menopause is critical for a smoother transition. With factual knowledge in your arsenal, you can face this life stage not with fear, but with understanding and a sense of control. Always remember that while menopause presents its challenges, it also opens the door to a new chapter filled with potential. It's a period of transformation that can be embraced with the right mindset, good health practices, and a supportive community.

Now that we've explored some of the myths and facts about menopause, you can step forward with confidence, knowing what to expect and what not to. Let this knowledge be the foundation on which you build your approach to managing mental health challenges during menopause, which we will delve into in the following chapters.

Chapter 2:
Recognizing Menopausal Mental Health Challenges

As we pivot from understanding the whirlwind of biological changes during menopause, it's crucial to illuminate the shadows of mental health challenges that may arise. This natural transition doesn't just signal a change in our bodies; it also brings about a transformation in our mental and emotional landscape. It's not uncommon to experience a cocktail of symptoms ranging from mood swings to a sense of melancholy. Maybe you're feeling a little more anxious than usual, or perhaps your mood takes a dip now and then. It's important to recognize these signals are part and parcel of the journey, not just a figment of your imagination or a reason to feel isolated. Acknowledging these challenges is the first step towards harnessing the tools and building the resilience needed to navigate this significant life stage with grace and empowerment. The following pages are dedicated to pulling these mental health threads into the light, unwinding the complexities, and presenting strategies that invite harmonious balance into your life during menopause.

Identifying Common Symptoms

As we traverse the menopausal landscape, it's paramount to familiarize ourselves with the variety of mental health challenges that can emerge. Understanding these symptoms is the first step towards managing them effectively. This journey is deeply personal, and every woman's experience is unique, yet certain commonalities bind us together.

Many women report a subtle onset of mood changes during this time. You might find yourself feeling irritable over the smallest things, or suddenly teary without a clear reason. These mood swings can be confusing, especially if you've always had a fairly even temperament. Remember, you're not alone in this; mood fluctuations are a common signpost along the menopausal road.

Another frequent visitor is anxiety, which can manifest in ways you might not immediately connect to menopause. Racing thoughts at 3 a.m., a heart pounding for no apparent reason, or a newfound sense of worry about day-to-day activities can all point to an anxiety symptom linked to the hormonal upheavals of menopause.

Don't overlook the more insidious symptom of depression. If you're feeling a persistent sadness, a loss of interest in activities you once enjoyed, or an unshakeable fatigue, it's worth discussing these feelings with a healthcare professional. It's easy to dismiss them as just an off day, but when they linger, they may be signaling something more significant.

Memory lapses and trouble concentrating can also come into play. While it's common to joke about "senior moments," there's nothing funny about the concern you might feel when you start forgetting names or tasks more frequently. This cognitive fog is often a side effect of the hormonal changes taking place in your body.

Let's talk about stress. Have you noticed that you're less resilient to life's stressors lately? Small inconveniences that you would have brushed off in the past now seem monumental. This diminished stress tolerance is your body's way of signaling that its coping mechanisms are currently under construction.

Then there's the feeling of being overwhelmed. Tasks that once seemed simple can appear daunting during menopause. These feelings are not a reflection of your abilities but rather a symptom of the transition you're navigating.

Some women also experience a shift in their self-esteem and self-image. Society's focus on youth can make the visible signs of aging tough to grapple with, and when these changes coincide with menopausal symptoms, it can be a recipe for feeling less confident in one's skin.

Sleep disturbances are another symptom that can exacerbate mental health challenges. If you're tossing and turning, struggling to get a good night's rest, you're certainly not alone. Sleep quality often diminishes during menopause, which can have a ripple effect on your overall mood and well-being.

Panic attacks are a less commonly discussed symptom of menopause, but for some women, they're a very real concern. The sudden onset of intense fear or discomfort, often accompanied by physical symptoms like a racing heart or shortness of breath, can be incredibly frightening.

Let's not forget the potential for paranoia or obsession. While less common than other symptoms, these can represent an extreme form of anxiety that can surface during this transitional period, causing significant distress.

Agitation and restlessness might start creeping into your days or nights. An inability to sit still or a persistent need to be busy can be signs of underlying menopausal anxiety, a signal that your body and mind are looking for outlets to cope with inner turmoil.

Feelings of disconnect or apathy can also be symptomatic of the menopausal transition. A sense of detachment from your surroundings or the people around you isn't uncommon. Your usual passions might not incite the same excitement, and this disinterest can be disconcerting.

Physical symptoms, too, like headaches, joint pain, or changes in libido, can have a substantial impact on mental health. These bodily experiences are deeply tied to our psychological state, and when your physical self doesn't feel right, it can throw your mental state out of balance.

Lastly, let's not minimize the potential onset of existential dread – questioning the meaning of life, your purpose, and your legacy can become especially prominent during this phase of life transition. It can feel daunting, but it's also a chance for deep personal growth and introspection.

As we move through these menopausal symptoms, it's vital to remain compassionate towards ourselves. Understanding these challenges paves the way toward seeking solutions and finding our balance once more. Don't hesitate to reach out for support; managing these symptoms is a critical step in maintaining your mental health and quality of life during and after the menopausal transition.

Depression, Anxiety, and Mood Swings

As we navigate the often choppy waters of menopause, it's vital to acknowledge that, yes, while hot flashes and night sweats are the talk of the town, the ebb and flow of our mental state is a cornerstone of this transition. Depression, anxiety, and mood swings can hit hard during menopause, sometimes making you feel like you're on an emotional roller coaster, sans the thrill. Estrogen isn't just about reproductive health; it's a key player in brain function, influencing mood and well-being, so when its levels dip, you might find yourself grappling with moodiness, sudden tears, or worrisome thoughts that you can't shake off. But let's take a breath and remember: you've navigated life's ups and downs before. This is just another bend in the river, and you're equipped with an oar called resilience. You're not alone on this journey, and recognizing these mental health challenges is the first, strong step towards managing them and reclaiming your joy. Let's ride this wave, arm ourselves with knowledge, and emerge stronger on the other side. Keep weaving that tapestry of well-being; it's a process, and every stitch counts.

The Role of Estrogen in Mental Health

Estrogen has been like a lifelong friend, intricately involved in so many facets of our health and well-being, especially within the neural corridors of our mental landscape. As we venture into understanding its role in mental health, particularly during menopause, we unearth a complexity that's both fascinating and vital for our journey.

Firstly, let's unravel the bond between estrogen and our brain. Estrogen isn't just about reproduction; it's a neuroprotective agent that guards the structure and function of the brain. Its influence sweeps across areas that govern mood, cognition, and even stress responses. But what happens when menopause ushers in a decline of this precious hormone?

For many, the decrease in estrogen can be like the dimming of lights at an ongoing party—things get a little less vivid, a bit moodier. There's a tangible connection between dropping estrogen levels and the roller coaster of emotions some may experience. It's not just fleeting sadness or transient worry—this hormonal shift can have a substantial impact on mental well-being.

Depression and anxiety, these familiar yet unwelcome guests, often knock louder at this stage of life. Estrogen's retreat has been linked to an increased susceptibility to these conditions. It's like the mind's weather pattern changes, with more frequent storms of mood swings appearing on the horizon.

The connection goes deeper. Neurotransmitters—the brain's chemical messengers—like serotonin and dopamine may also dance to the tune of estrogen. As the levels of this hormone wane, these neurotransmitters' functioning can be thrown off balance, sometimes triggering depressive symptoms or anxiety. It's an intricate dance indeed, with every dip and rise holding significant sway over our mental state.

Remember though, you're not at the mercy of these hormonal shifts. There's empowerment in knowledge and taking action. Lifestyle adjustments can rekindle the light that estrogen dims. From nutritional tweaks to exercise, the keys to unlock a more stable mood lie within your reach.

Cognitive functions, too—such as memory and focus—can feel the impact of estrogen's decline. Some of you might notice a slight fog setting in, a consequence of this hormonal shift. It's vital to recognize these changes as potential signs of menopausal transition, rather than an irreversible decline in mental faculties.

Why does all this matter? Because it frames our experience, it shapes the narrative of our transition through menopause. When we understand the roots of our emotional ebbs and flows, we equip ourselves to navigate them with grace and resilience.

Sleep, dear friends, is another realm under estrogen's reign that can be disrupted. As the levels dip, insomnia can become a familiar foe, leading to fatigue which, in a cruel twist, can exacerbate mood disturbances and cognitive challenges. Appreciate the interconnectedness of these experiences; they don't stand alone but rather weave together in the tapestry of menopausal transition.

What can be done? Well, stepping into the light of self-care and actively seeking supportive strategies can be transformative. Regular exercise isn't just about physical health; it's a natural buoy for mental health, boosting those endorphins that lift the spirits and clearing the cobwebs from the mind.

As estrogen takes a step back, don't hesitate to reach out for support. Therapy, whether it be talk therapy, cognitive-behavioral therapy, or other forms, can provide tools to manage these hormonal fluctuations with more finesse and less distress.

There's also hope in the form of hormone replacement therapy (HRT), where appropriate and under professional supervision. It can serve as a bridge over troubled waters for some, replenishing the estrogen that's slipped away, and potentially easing the mental health challenges of menopause.

But, let's not forget the might of mindfulness and meditation—practices that fortify the mind's resilience. They remind us that while we can't control the hormonal waves, we can learn to surf them with a steadiness that comes from within.

Nutrition plays its part too, offering up natural sources of phytoestrogens or foods rich in Omega-3 fatty acids that support mental health. It's like discovering a map to hidden treasures within the realm of our diet, treasures that can ease this transitional journey.

Lastly, as we walk through this chapter of life, let's weave a narrative of empowerment rather than one of loss. Yes, the role of estrogen in mental health is complex and deeply significant, but it doesn't write our entire story. Our mental tapestry can still burst with vibrant hues, threaded with the wisdom, self-care, and support that we weave into our days. The journey through menopause is not just a physiological one; it's a passage ripe for growth, ripe for us to emerge wiser, stronger, and grounded in the fullness of who we are.

Chapter 3:
The Power of Positive Thinking

Transitioning right into the heart of our conversation, let's talk about a tool you already possess that can be more potent than any supplement or medication: your mindset. Positive thinking doesn't mean ignoring life's less pleasant situations. It's about approaching the challenges of menopause with a more optimistic and proactive standpoint. It's a known fact that the way we think—our internal dialogue—has a tremendous impact on how we feel both physically and emotionally. By nurturing a hopeful outlook, you're not simply donning rose-colored glasses; you're actively constructing a framework that can support mental resilience throughout menopause and beyond. Remember, you've navigated life's ups and downs before, and this transition is yet another phase where your inner strength can shine. Cultivating positivity isn't about perfection—it's about embracing the flux, learning to reframe thoughts and expectations, and recognizing that while the road might have its bumps, you have the grace and grit to travel it with your head held high.

Cultivating a Positive Mindset

Navigating the waters of menopause can feel overwhelming, but planting the seeds of positivity in your daily mindset can blossom into powerful change. It starts with acknowledging that your thoughts hold immense sway over your emotions and body. By consciously steering your mind towards the good—a compliment from a friend, the peacefulness of your morning coffee; the warmth of the sun on your skin—you fuel resilience against the tide of hormonal shifts. It's about celebrating the small wins, like choosing salad over fries or finally tackling that cluttered closet, because these victories add richness and color to the fabric of your day. Remember, it's not about being relentlessly upbeat but about finding balance. By gently nudging away from self-criticism and embracing a more compassionate inner dialogue, you'll find that the challenges of menopause aren't just manageable—they're a platform for growth and rejuvenation.

Reframing Thoughts and Expectations

Transitioning through menopause can often feel like navigating through a maze without a map. It's a time of physical change, sure, but it's the shifts in our mindset and expectations that can dramatically influence our experience. The good news is that by actively reframing our thoughts and expectations, we can journey through this natural stage of life not just with resilience, but with a sense of empowerment.

Our thoughts are powerful; they can be our greatest allies or our most critical adversaries. The key is learning the art of cognitive reframing—a tool that can transform our mental landscape during the menopausal transition. Instead of viewing hot flashes as an inevitable misery, for instance, we might see them as signals to slow down and practice self-care. While this doesn't diminish the discomfort, it shifts our perception to a space where we can respond rather than react.

Expectations about menopause are often steeped in cultural narratives that focus on loss—the end of fertility, the decline of youth. However, by reframing this transition as a beginning rather than an ending, we unlock a new narrative. This is a period rich with opportunity for personal growth, a sort of coming-of-age that happens at a later stage in life, where wisdom is the coveted trait, not just youthful vigor.

Let's discuss the whispers of ageism, the subtle and not-so-subtle messages suggesting that with menopause comes irrelevance. By challenging these myths and altering our internal script, we can embrace a new self-identity that celebrates the insights and experience unique to this phase of life. Imagine replacing 'I am becoming older and less significant' with 'I am evolving into a more nuanced and assertive version of myself.'

Menopause doesn't come with a universal playbook because everyone's experience is distinctly their own. What worked for a friend may not work for you. By staying open to a personalized journey, while learning from others, you can set expectations that align with your individual needs and lifestyle. This approach empowers you to find what truly works for you, rather than fitting into a one-size-fits-all mold.

It's also essential to reframe the expectation that menopause is a static state; it's anything but. Like all of life, it's a dynamic process with ebbs and flows. There will be good days and challenging ones—anticipating this can prepare us to ride the waves with grace and adapt strategies as needed. Flexibility becomes our strength, not a concession to unpredictability.

Another vital aspect of reframing involves the reshaping of our social lives. Menopause might coincide with children leaving home or relationships evolving. Instead of mourning these shifts, try reframing them as an invitation to explore new interests and deepen existing relationships—or cultivate new ones. This is a time when companionship can take on new forms, providing a support system that reflects who you are now.

How we frame our conversations about menopause, both with ourselves and with others, profoundly impacts our psyche. Choosing language that's empowering and accurate can dismantle the stigma and promote a healthier dialogue. For instance, talking about 'surviving' menopause feels very different from discussing 'thriving' through it. Language is the brush we use to paint our personal narratives, so we might as well pick colors that uplift and inspire.

We ought to address the unease we might feel about physical changes—here lies an opportunity for profound reframing. Can we view these changes as marks of a life fully lived rather than signs of decline? Embracing our evolving bodies as testaments to our journey is a radical act of self-love that redefines beauty standards on our terms, opening up a path toward self-acceptance that is both liberating and invigorating.

Reframing can also extend to how we manage symptoms. Instead of a narrow focus on the discomforts, we can create a broader picture that includes proactive management. For example, rather than dreading sleep disruptions, we could see bedtime as a chance to indulge in relaxing routines or explore strategies like mindful breathing that enhance sleep quality while enriching our overall well-being.

When it comes to the emotional waves, often amplified by hormonal fluctuations, there's scope to reframe these too. Rather than pathologizing every mood swing, we can acknowledge that emotions are messengers offering insights into our needs. This perspective encourages us to listen and respond with self-compassion rather than judgment, nurturing our emotional landscape.

Menopause also invites a reframing of our professional lives. Instead of fearing a decline in productivity or relevance, we might see this as a season to leverage our seasoned expertise or pivot toward new ventures that have been on the backburner. It's a chance to redefine success on our own matured terms, embracing the skills and insights honed over years of experience.

Lastly, when setting health goals during menopause, it's important to reframe our expectations about progress. Rather than adhere to rigid benchmarks, consider setting intentions that honor the body's changing rhythms and needs. This might include integrating gentle forms of exercise, prioritizing recovery, and celebrating each small victory on the path to well-being.

Reframing thoughts and expectations is not about dismissing the realities of menopause, but rather about claiming agency over the narrative. It's a powerful and ongoing practice that can transform challenges into chapters of adaptation, growth, and empowerment in our life stories. And in this process, we become not just survivors of menopause but pioneers of a new, richly textured stage of life.

As we move forward, let's remember that the way we think about our experiences is just as crucial as the experiences themselves. Reframing doesn't happen overnight—it's a commitment to a continuously evolving mindset. But with each step, each shift in perspective, we're not just getting through menopause; we're reshaping it into a journey that reflects the fullness of who we are and all that we have yet to become.

Chapter 4:
Managing Stress and Anxiety

As we journey deeper into the heart of menopause, let's take a moment to acknowledge a common travel companion: stress. Now, rather than letting it snag our spirits, imagine embracing stress as a signal, a nudge pointing us towards nurturing our inner balance. In this chapter, we're diving into a world where mindfulness is our anchor and relaxation isn't just a luxury; it's essential. We'll learn to ride the waves of anxiety with the finesse of a seasoned surfer, controlling our breath and centering our thoughts. Anxiety, that tricky beast, often feels like a maze with no exit, but picture yourself as the architect of that maze. You can dismantle it, one calming breath, one mindful moment at a time. You're not alone in this, and the tools you'll discover here are like keys to unlock a more serene state of mind, despite the hormonal hustle. Tune into your body's wisdom—it's there, even if the signals seem a little scrambled at times—and trust that you'll find clarity amid the chaos. You've got this, and this chapter is here to guide you through unfurling the sails of serenity in your menopausal voyage.

Mindfulness and Relaxation Techniques

As you navigate the often tumultuous waters of menopause, it's essential to anchor yourself with effective stress-management strategies. Mindfulness and relaxation techniques can be your invaluable allies on this journey. While it's common to feel overwhelmed by the physiological and emotional changes during this time, shifting your focus inward and harnessing the power of the present moment can work wonders. Delving into practices like guided imagery or progressive muscle relaxation not only eases the mind but helps to cultivate a state of calm amidst the storm. Embrace these practices as personal rituals to foster inner tranquility and resilience. Such techniques are more than mere stress-busters; they're invitations to rediscover serenity, empowering you to embrace each day with renewed calmness and clarity. Remember, nurturing your mental oasis isn't an indulgence — it's a vital part of your health during menopause and beyond.

Breathing Exercises and Meditation can become formidable allies in your journey through menopause. Amidst all the unexpected waves of change, these practices offer a stable, soothing anchor— turning turmoil into tranquility. Here we'll explore profound, yet simple techniques designed to fend off anxiety, and to nurture a calm, centered state of mind.

Let's start with the basics: your breath is a powerful tool. It's free, always accessible, and remarkably under your control. Breathing exercises can have immediate effects on decreasing stress hormones, slowing down your heart rate, and lowering blood pressure. One popular technique is diaphragmatic breathing, or deep belly breathing, which involves fully engaging your diaphragm and expanding your lungs.

Try it out—we'll do it together. Get comfortable, either sitting or lying down. Place one hand on your chest and the other on your belly. Inhale slowly through your nose, feeling your stomach push your hand up. Keep your chest still. Then exhale through your mouth as your stomach falls. Repeat this pattern, establishing a slow, rhythmic flow. The beautiful thing about deep belly breathing is its simplicity. It's as though you're giving your body a mini vacation—a few moments of pure relaxation.

Moving beyond the belly, we can also integrate techniques that target the rhythm and length of your breath. Paced Respiration—a method specifically beneficial during hot flashes—involves slow, deep breathing at a rate of around 5 to 7 breaths per minute. Such measured breathing can reduce the frequency of hot flashes and create a sense of cool composure. As with any skill, the key to mastery is consistent practice; these breathing exercises are no different.

Meditation, the sister strategy of breathing exercises, ushers in a multitude of mental health benefits. It's like a gentle workout for your mind—building strength, flexibility, and resilience. Don't worry if you're new to this; meditation doesn't demand hours of your day. Even short periods can be significantly impactful.

There are various forms of meditation, each with its unique focus and benefits. Mindfulness meditation, for instance, emphasizes the art of being present. It teaches you to observe your thoughts and emotions without judgment, to simply be aware of them as they come and go. This form of meditation can be particularly useful during menopause, a time when your mind might seem like it's operating on a tempestuous sea. Mindfulness brings the calm, allowing you to navigate your thoughts with grace and patience.

Another form that can be quite soothing is guided visualization. Here, you transport yourself mentally to a peaceful setting—a sun-drenched beach, a tranquil forest, or a serene mountaintop. These guided journeys can provide respite from the stress and anxiety that often accompany menopause.

Loving-kindness meditation is another transformative practice. It involves directing positive energy and well wishes to yourself and others. It can fuel feelings of compassion and connection, counteracting the sense of isolation or the challenges of mood swings that may arise during this phase of life.

Maybe you're thinking, "That all sounds fine, but how do I begin?" It's simple: start where you are. There's no need for special equipment or a picturesque setting. Just find a quiet spot, perhaps even the same one where you perform your breathing exercises. Start with a couple of minutes each day, and as you grow more comfortable, gradually extend your sessions. Commitment and patience are your true companions here. Don't be discouraged if your mind seems too busy at first—that's completely normal, and it will settle with time.

As you explore these exercises, remember, it's not about perfection. It's about progress and personal growth. Each breath you take is an opportunity to bring yourself back to a state of balance—to harness control amidst the whirlwind of hot flashes, sleep disturbances, and emotional rollercoasters.

A fascinating aspect of breathing exercises and meditation is the research supporting their effects on the brain. Studies have shown that these practices can change your brain's structure and function in ways that promote emotional well-being and cognitive health. In times when you may feel at the mercy of your fluctuating hormones, meditation and controlled breathing can help you reclaim agency over your mental state.

Moreover, these practices dovetail beautifully with positive thinking strategies and relaxation techniques discussed in previous chapters. By integrating them into your routine, you create a potent synergy—a lifestyle that continuously feeds into your mental and emotional wellness.

It's also vital to recognize that while meditation and breathing exercises can significantly aid in managing mental health challenges during menopause, they don't replace professional help if needed. They are part of a holistic approach, one facet of a multi-dimensional plan encompassing nutrition, physical activity, social connections, and possibly even hormone therapy.

We've laid a lot of information before you, but don't let it overwhelm you. Start small, stay consistent, and be patient. Incorporate these practices into your daily routine, tailor them to your needs, and observe the changes. You may just find that breathing exercises and meditation become your most cherished tools in riding out the waves of menopause with serenity and strength.

Chapter 5:
Nurturing Your Emotional Well-being

As you turn the page on stress and anxiety management, isn't it time we explore the lush gardens of emotional well-being? Now, menopause isn't just a physical roller coaster—it's an emotional odyssey, replete with its highs and lows. As you meander through these changes, it's vital to anchor yourself, learning to express emotions in a way that's both healthy and liberating. Consider this chapter your personal toolkit for emotional resilience. It's about cloaking yourself in understanding and kindness as you navigate the choppy waters of mood fluctuations. Let's carve out spaces for those heartfelt dialogues and cultivate inner strength. It's about standing in the midst of a hormonal whirlwind and saying, "I've got this," because you know what? You truly do. Together, we will layer the foundations of a robust emotional well-being, ensuring that as your body adapts to a new normal, your spirit remains unshakable, radiant, and ever so resilient.

Emotional Expression and Menopause

As you journey through the ripples and waves of menopause, there's an often understated yet vital element that deserves our focus: the art of emotional expression. You've probably noticed that your emotions can be akin to a rollercoaster during this transitional phase. It's not just you – many women experience a wide spectrum of feelings due to the hormonal changes that menopause ushers in.

Estrogen and progesterone, those key hormonal players, aren't just about physical symptoms; they impact your brain, too. When their levels start to dance to a different tune, your emotions might also start swinging to a chaotic rhythm. It's perfectly normal—and acknowledging this is the first step to nurturing your emotional well-being.

One day you might be feeling sharp as a tack, and the next, you could be engulfed in a fog of sadness or irritation. Remember that it's okay to feel this way. Emotional expression is not a sign of weakness; it's a profound display of your humanity and it's as essential as breathing. The trick, they say, is not to let those feelings define you or take the reins of your day-to-day life.

Let's talk about strategies to express and manage your emotions. Journaling can be incredibly therapeutic. It doesn't have to be a meticulous daily diary—sometimes just scribbling your thoughts on a notepad can help untangle them. Seeing your feelings on paper can lend perspective and make them seem more manageable.

Another key strategy is communication. Talking with friends, family, or a support group about what you're experiencing can provide relief and a sense of belonging. You're not alone. There are numerous women navigating the same tumultuous seas of menopause, and sharing your journey can help lighten the load.

When intense feelings surge up, don't underestimate the power of creative outlets. Art, music, dance, or whatever form of creativity that speaks to you can serve as a potent form of emotional expression. Engaging in these activities can provide a much-needed escape valve for bottled-up emotions.

It's also essential to maintain a sense of humor about the craziness of it all. Sometimes, a good laugh over the more absurd moments is more therapeutic than we give it credit for. Find humor in the everyday and let it act as your companion through the peaks and valleys of menopause.

Be mindful of the emotional traps that can ensnare you when you're feeling vulnerable. It's easy to slip into a pattern of negative thinking or to start catastrophizing. When you catch yourself spiraling down these paths, press pause. Take a deep breath, and gently guide your thoughts back to a kinder, more balanced perspective.

Mindfulness and relaxation techniques aren't just for bodily relaxation—they're also champions of emotional composure. Whether it's through yoga, meditation, or simple breathing exercises, making space for tranquility in your life can provide the emotional equipoise you long for.

Don't shy away from seeking professional help if you find that your emotions become overwhelming. Therapists are like navigators in the often stormy ocean of menopause. They can help you understand and work through your feelings with professional tools and strategies tailored just for you.

Self-expression doesn't always have to be about revealing your pain or frustrations. It can also be about celebrating your victories, no matter how small they may seem. Every step you take in understanding and expressing your emotions is a win—so give yourself some credit for that.

Apart from hormonal changes, your life experiences and stressors add another layer to your emotional canvas. Menopause might coincide with other significant life changes like children leaving home, aging parents, or career transitions. Recognizing how these factors can compound emotional challenges is important for navigating them more effectively.

While you're tackling the woes of menopause, remember to foster a sense of resilience. You've overcome a multitude of challenges throughout your life, and this is another chapter you'll conquer. Cultivating an unyielding spirit amidst the chaos will fuel your journey to emotional balance and well-being.

Finally, practicing self-compassion is non-negotiable. Be gentle with yourself. Understand that it's normal to have an off day—or days—as you traverse menopause. Extending the same compassion and understanding to yourself that you would offer a dear friend makes a world of difference in your mental and emotional health.

Remember, the fluctuations of the heart and mind you're experiencing are transient and wholly valid. They're signposts on your journey, not your final destination. By embracing and expressing your emotions, you'll not only survive the menopausal transition, you'll emerge with a renewed sense of self and strength. Hold onto this belief as we delve further into building emotional resilience, which is another cornerstone in nurturing your emotional well-being.

Building Emotional Resilience

The journey through menopause is one that's unique to every woman, filled with not just physical changes but emotional ones as well. It's during these times of transition where building emotional resilience becomes a quintessential skill to navigate the choppy waters. Emotional resilience doesn't mean you won't experience stress, sadness, or anxiety. What resilience does is contribute to your ability to bounce back from those challenges stronger and more adaptable.

First, let's tackle the idea of acceptance. Accepting that the menopausal transition is a normal part of life can be liberating. Your body is not betraying you; it's simply moving into a new phase. By welcoming this phase, we set the stage for emotional resilience. This acceptance allows you to address the changes head-on rather than resisting what seems like an unyielding tide.

Another cornerstone of emotional resilience is maintaining a balanced perspective. It's easy to get fixated on the negatives, especially when symptoms can feel overwhelming. However, focusing on the positives can not only lift your mood but also reduce stress. Perhaps you've noticed a new sense of freedom or an opportunity to focus more on personal growth. Whatever your silver lining is, holding onto it can make a significant difference on tough days.

Stress management is also critical. Chronic stress can exacerbate menopausal symptoms like hot flashes and disrupt your sleep. Try incorporating mindfulness exercises into your daily routine. Just a few minutes of mindful breathing or meditation each day can help lower stress levels and improve your emotional well-being. When we consciously direct our attention to the present moment, we often find that our stresses are either manageable or not as intense as we perceived them to be.

It's also important to develop a strong network of support. Surround yourself with friends, family, or a community that understands what you're going through. Sharing experiences can not only provide relief but can also help you gather new strategies for managing symptoms. A strong support system is a safety net, offering a sense of security and belonging during times of change.

Physical health plays a role in emotional resilience, too. Regular exercise, a balanced diet, and adequate sleep are all foundational elements of mental health. When the body feels good, the mind often follows. Find activities you enjoy, foods that nourish, and strive for a restful night's sleep to keep your emotional resilience strong.

Next, let's talk about coping strategies. Menopause can be an emotional rollercoaster, so having a toolkit of coping mechanisms is vital. This may include journaling, engaging in a hobby, or practicing yoga. These activities offer an outlet for stress and serve as a reminder that you have control over your well-being.

Learning when to say "no" is another aspect of building resilience. You don't have to do everything for everyone. Setting boundaries is about protecting your energy and prioritizing your needs. Remember, self-care isn't selfish; it's essential.

It's also beneficial to develop a practice of self-compassion. Being kind to yourself during moments of struggle is a form of emotional first aid. Understand that it's okay to have a mix of good and bad days and acknowledge your feelings without judgment. Show yourself the same compassion that you would offer a dear friend.

Strengthening your problem-solving skills can help you approach menopausal challenges with confidence. Instead of viewing symptoms as insurmountable obstacles, see them as problems that can be worked through or managed. Whether it's brainstorming solutions for sleep disturbances or developing strategies to handle mood swings, each successful problem solved reinforces your ability to cope.

Don't underestimate the power of humor. Finding humor in life's ups and downs is a sign of emotional strength. Laughter can boost your mood, relieve stress, and even improve your immune system. So, indulge in your favorite comedy or share a joke with a friend—it's good for your resilience quotient.

Embrace new opportunities for personal growth. Menopause might signify the end of a certain bodily function, but it can also be the beginning of newfound interests or passions. This phase can be a perfect time to reevaluate your priorities and embark on new projects.

Remember, resilience is not about never falling; it's about learning how to get back up. If you're struggling with a particularly difficult symptom, seek help. Whether it's speaking to a therapist, consulting your doctor, or joining a support group, taking action is a step towards resilience.

It's also helpful to create a vision for your life post-menopause. This can be an inspiring incentive to manage your emotional health during the menopausal transition. Visualize how you want to feel and what you want to achieve. This future-focused outlook can provide motivation and hope.

Lastly, document your journey. Write down your experiences, your feelings, and your triumphs. This record not only serves as a reminder of how far you've come but also reinforces the positive coping strategies that work for you. Reviewing this personal narrative can give you a burst of resilience on days when you need it the most.

Building emotional resilience is a process that doesn't happen overnight, but every step you take strengthens your ability to handle the menopausal transition with grace and confidence. By cultivating resilience, you're not just surviving menopause; you're thriving through it. Let each triumph, no matter how small, be a stepping stone to a more emotionally resilient you.

Chapter 6:
Sleep Solutions for Menopausal Women

After learning about nurturing your emotional well-being, it's time we turn our focus onto one of the most common battles you might be facing: sleep disruptions. Tossing and turning throughout the night can become the norm, but it certainly doesn't have to be your reality. Sleep is crucial, especially now, as your body navigates the complexities of menopause, affecting everything from your mood to your cognitive function. Let's dive into some practical and empowering strategies to reclaim those precious hours of rest. You'll find that a few changes to your evening routine or sleeping environment might just be the key to unlocking the rejuvenating, restful slumber you deserve. Remember that you're not alone in this; countless women have stood where you're standing and have found ways to overcome these nocturnal nuisances. So together, let's explore these pathways, not just to better sleep, but to a brighter, more energetic tomorrow.

Understanding Sleep Disruptions

As we navigate the menopausal labyrinth, it becomes abundantly clear that sleep, the gentle restorer, sometimes turns into a nightly puzzle that just doesn't seem to fit together like it used to. Those midnight awakenings, they're not just a fluke; they're rooted in the shifting sands of our hormonal landscape. Think of estrogen as a conductor of an orchestra, ensuring all parts play in harmony. When its levels drop, the symphony of our body's functions can experience discordance. Hot flashes are the infamous culprits, notorious for their unpredictability and intensity, often searing through our sleep. Then there's the sleep architecture itself, remodeling during menopause like a house undergoing renovation, with less time in the deep, restorative stages of sleep, making it feel as though rest is just a veneer over the surface of tiredness. While we can't turn back the hands of time to reclaim the hormone levels of our youth, we're not relegated to endless nights of tossing and turning. Understanding these disruptions is the cornerstone upon which we can build a fortress of strategies to reclaim the night and awaken refreshed and ready to embrace the day with open arms and a rested mind.

Strategies for Improved Sleep Quality Through the menopausal transition, deciphering the puzzle of sleep can feel like a nightly battle. You're not alone if you find yourself tossing, turning, and looking at the clock as it ticks away precious moments of rest. Quality sleep is not a luxury; it's a necessity, especially during this unique period of life.

Let's start by emphasizing the importance of a consistent sleep schedule. Our bodies thrive on routine, and by going to bed and waking up at the same time every day, we can reinforce our natural circadian rhythms. Yes, even on weekends! This regularity can help ease those disruptive night wakings and make the slide into sleep smoother and sweeter.

Creating a serene sleep environment is also paramount. The bedroom should be a sanctuary, reserved exclusively for sleep and intimacy. This means keeping work-related materials, electronics, and other distractions at bay. Invest in comfort with a supportive mattress, plush pillows, and soft, breathable bedding. You're crafting a nest that cradles you into slumber, separating the day's stress from the night's peace.

Consider the role of temperature too. Our body temperature drops as we fall asleep, so a cool room can significantly support this natural process. Keeping the thermostat set to a comfortable, cooler setting can create an ideal climate for drifting off. Pair this with moisture-wicking sleepwear, especially designed for those experiencing night sweats, and you've got a dynamic duo for a cooler night's rest.

The power of darkness should not be underestimated. Melatonin, our sleep hormone, is influenced by light exposure. Use heavy curtains or a sleep mask to block out light, and steer clear of bright screens at least an hour before bedtime. This includes your phone, tablet, and television. Instead, dim the lights and engage in a tranquil activity like reading or listening to calming music.

Magnesium-rich foods can be a sleep-friendly addition to your diet. Think leafy greens, nuts, seeds, and whole grains. These aren't just nutritious choices; they can also promote relaxation. Some find that a small snack high in protein before bed can keep nighttime hunger pangs from disrupting sleep without weighing down the digestive system.

Caffeine and alcohol deserve a second look when it comes to their impact on sleep. Both substances can interfere with the ability to fall and stay asleep, with effects that can last hours after consumption. Try to limit intake of these stimulants, particularly in the second half of the day when they can wreak havoc on your bedtime routine.

Physical activity is an ally for good sleep, as long as it's not too close to bedtime. Exercise can improve the duration and quality of sleep by promoting the release of endorphins and reducing stress. However, engaging in vigorous activity late in the evening can be too stimulating. Aim to wrap up workouts at least three hours before you plan to hit the hay.

There's also room to incorporate mindfulness and relaxation techniques into your pre-bedtime routine. Gentle yoga, deep-breathing exercises, or progressive muscle relaxation can lower stress levels and prepare the mind and body for sleep. These practices soothe the transition from the busyness of the day into the stillness of the night.

An often overlooked aspect is proper hydration. Dehydration can lead to discomfort and frequent awakenings, yet too much fluid before bedtime can lead to disruptive nocturnal trips to the bathroom. Strike a balance by drinking ample fluids throughout the day, tapering off as the evening progresses.

Naps, while refreshing, can be a double-edged sword. If you must indulge in a daytime snooze, keep it brief and early in the afternoon. Short power naps can recharge you without stealing from your nighttime sleep currency. Aim for 20 minutes – long enough for a rest but not so long that it leaves you groggy or affects your ability to fall asleep later.

For some, natural sleep aids such as melatonin supplements, valerian root, or chamomile tea can gently coax the body toward sleep. However, it's wise to consult with a healthcare professional before adding any supplements to your routine, ensuring they're appropriate for your unique health profile and won't interact with other medications.

A lesser-known trick is to utilize the bed for sleep association. If you're lying awake for over 20 minutes, get up and engage in a calming activity elsewhere before trying to sleep again. This technique prevents your brain from associating the bed with frustration and wakefulness, making it more likely that you'll fall asleep upon your return.

And let's not forget journaling. Sometimes, racing thoughts can be the biggest barrier to sleep. Keeping a journal by your bed to jot down worries or to-do lists can clear your mind, helping you let go of the day's concerns, trusting that they will be there in the morning after a restorative night of rest.

Lastly, remember that the quality of your daytime hours affects the quality of your nighttime rest. Engaging in stress-reducing activities, maintaining social connections, and finding joy in hobbies can reduce the mental clutter that often bubbles up when our heads hit the pillow.

Implementing just a few of these strategies can make a considerable difference in your sleep quality. It's about creating a personalized recipe for rest, one that acknowledges and respects the unique shifts occurring within your body during menopause. With patience and a willingness to experiment, you can reclaim the night and the myriad of benefits that come with a good night's sleep. Sweet dreams!

Chapter 7: Nutrition for the Mind

As we've embraced the transformative journey of menopause and explored the terrain of mental well-being, let's nourish our brains with the same gusto that we apply to tending our gardens. Now, imagine your mind as a fertile landscape where the right nutrients can bloom into a state of cognitive clarity and emotional stability. In this favored chapter, 'Nutrition for the Mind,' we're going to delve into the culinary symphony of brain-boosting fare that supports our thinking, lifts our spirits, and fortifies our mental acumen during the menopausal transition. I'm talking about vibrant omega-3 rich salmons swimming upstream in your diet, plump blueberries bursting with antioxidants, and the aromatic spices like turmeric sprinkled in for their anti-inflammatory prowess. We'll uncover how a tapestry of whole foods is not only a feast for our senses but also a catalyst for maintaining, and even improving, our cognitive health. Moreover, we'll sift through the labyrinth of supplements, demystifying which can be the allies in our quest for mental acuteness. Let's transform our kitchens into havens of brain health, one delicious, nutrient-dense bite at a time.

Brain-Boosting Foods

Navigating the menopausal journey can sometimes feel like traversing a cognitive labyrinth, but fear not, certain foods can serve as a reliable compass. You're well aware of the potent power of nutrition when it comes to managing your physical health, but what about sustaining and nourishing your mind? Let's dive into the culinary allies that can sharpen your wit and soften the fog. Incorporate fatty fish rich in omega-3s, such as salmon and mackerel, to bolster cell membranes in your brain and support neurological function. Antioxidant-packed berries help in warding off oxidative stress, which is just as critical for brain cells as it is for skin cells. Leafy greens, thanks to their high folate and vitamins, can provide a buffer against cognitive decline. In addition to these, there's a whole repertoire, from nuts like walnuts that resemble little brains for a reason, to glorious dark chocolate that not only satisfies your taste buds but also contains flavonoids to fire up your neuron activity. Embrace these nutrient-dense champions in your diet and you might just find your thoughts as agile and vibrant as your nourished, menopause-powered spirit.

Supplements for Cognitive Health Continuing our journey through the nourishment of the mind during menopause, let's dive into the world of supplements and how they can support our cognitive health. It's no secret that as women transit through menopause, some may notice changes in their memory or cognitive abilities. While these can sometimes be worrisome, there are several supplements on the market that just might boost your brain power. But remember, it's crucial to discuss with your healthcare provider before starting any new supplement regimen.

First on our list is Omega-3 fatty acids, known for their role in brain health. These are essential fats found in high quantities in fish oil, which studies suggest can help maintain memory and cognitive function. The brain loves these fats, and they can combat inflammation – a key factor in cognitive decline. Consider incorporating omega-3s through diet or high-quality supplements.

Another powerful player is Vitamin D – the "sunshine vitamin." This nutrient is vital for bone health, yes, but it also has a part to play in our cognitive realm. Some research links Vitamin D deficiency to a higher risk of cognitive decline. Since getting enough from sunlight alone can be challenging, especially during the winter months, a supplement could be your beam of intellectual light.

Curcumin, the active ingredient in the spice turmeric, has a reputation for being a potent anti-inflammatory and antioxidant.

Some studies propose that it may also aid in boosting brain-derived neurotrophic factor (BDNF), which could support brain health. A sprinkle of turmeric in your meals or a curcumin supplement might just be your golden ticket.

Ginkgo biloba is an ancient herb, and its leaves are used in supplements to possibly help with cognitive function. The argument is that it improves blood flow to the brain, thus enhancing brain activity. Research has been mixed, so it's not a sure bet, but it may be worth exploring if you're interested in herbal options.

The antioxidant properties of Vitamin E have been theorized to protect cells from damage, including those of the brain. It's said that a little vitamin E boost might go a long way in maintaining cognitive function as you age. However, be mindful of the dosage, as high levels can carry risks.

B vitamins, particularly B6, B9 (folate), and B12, are important for overall brain health. They play a role in reducing homocysteine levels, high levels of which are associated with cognitive decline and dementia. Keeping up with B's could help keep the mind sharp, but again, moderation is key, and it's wise to seek guidance from a healthcare provider.

Acetyl-L-carnitine, an amino acid naturally produced in the body, is thought to benefit brain health by providing energy to the brain and supporting the health of brain cells. For those going through menopause, a supplement could potentially be a helping hand for mental clarity and energy levels.

Magnesium, which plays an important part in many different brain functions, is another mineral at which to take a closer look. Magnesium threonate, in particular, may have the ability to cross the blood-brain barrier and enhance learning and memory functions. Be sure to check with your doctor to determine the right type and dose of magnesium for you.

Resveratrol, the compound often heralded for its presence in red wine, has also been investigated for its potential brain-boosting benefits. As an antioxidant and anti-inflammatory agent, it could help slow down age-related cognitive decline. But moderation is wise - while a little may be helpful, it's not an invitation to overindulge.

Phosphatidylserine, a fat compound called a phospholipid which covers and protects cells in your brain, has been associated with preserving memory and preventing cognitive decline. Although the body makes this compound, levels can decline with age. Therefore, supplementation could be a smart move.

For those grappling with brain fog and a lapse in concentration, L-Theanine – an amino acid primarily found in tea leaves – could provide some mental clarity. Well-known for promoting relaxation without drowsiness, it's often combined with caffeine for an enhanced cognitive boost.

Then there's Bacopa monnieri, an herb traditionally used in Ayurvedic medicine to improve brain function. It's been suggested to enhance learning and memory and reduce anxiety – something that could be particularly beneficial for women in menopause experiencing cognitive concerns.

As we explore these supplements, it's essential to remember that they are just that – supplements. None are magic bullets, and they should complement a healthy lifestyle that includes balanced nutrition, ample sleep, regular physical activity, and stress management techniques. Incorporate them as part of a holistic approach to your menopausal wellness plan.

Lastly, let's not forget to address safety. Just because supplements are available over the counter doesn't mean they're harmless. Some can interact with medications, or may not be suitable given a person's health history. That's why it's so important to have a chat with your healthcare provider to ensure the best path for your health and cognitive well-being.

In sum, supplements could potentially support cognitive health during menopause, but they should be used judiciously. And always, they must be part of a broader, comprehensive approach that values the connection between physical, mental, and emotional health. Let's keep our brains just as nourished as our bodies as we navigate this transformative stage of life.

Chapter 8:
The Importance of Physical Activity

As we pivot from the critical role nutrition plays in maintaining mental health during menopause, let's not overlook the transformative power of physical activity. You've likely heard it a million times: exercise is vital for your health. But in the midst of the menopausal transition, its benefits are amplified tenfold. Movement isn't just about keeping the scales at bay or maintaining a certain dress size—it's a proven mood lifter and stress reducer that can sharpen your mental clarity amidst the fog of fluctuating hormones. Think of exercise as a natural elixir; it's capable of coaxing endorphins to the surface, offering that blissful 'runner's high' without pounding the pavement for miles. Whether it's dancing in your living room, joining a yoga class, or simply taking a brisk walk, finding an activity you love can be the game-changer in your mental health toolkit. And it's not a one-size-fits-all; your body, your rules. So let's lace up those sneakers and delve into how syncing up your workouts with your wellness goals can clear the mind, lift spirits, and empower you through this season of change.

Exercise and Mental Clarity

As you embrace the transformative period of menopause, integrating physical activity into your life is like a breath of fresh air for your mind. The endorphins released during exercise don't just elevate your mood; they clear the mental fog that can cloak your thoughts during menopausal transitions. Whether you're dancing to your favorite tunes or taking a brisk walk in nature, these movements dilute the stresses that may have crystallized over the day, enhancing your focus and cognitive sharpness. It's empowering to witness how lacing up those sneakers for a jog or unfolding your yoga mat can unravel the tangles of your thoughts and set the stage for clearer, more vibrant mental landscapes. Trust in the rhythmic beat of your heart and the strength in your muscles to guide you toward mental clarity and an invigorated spirit, allowing the pieces of your day to fall into place with a newfound ease.

Tailoring Your Workout Regimen is an empowering step in your journey through menopause. It's not just about staying fit; it's about shaping an exercise routine that resonates with your body's unique needs during this time of change. Gone are the days of one-size-fits-all fitness plans. Your body is going through a metamorphosis, and it's only fitting that your workouts do the same.

First, let's acknowledge the elephant in the room: fatigue. It's common to feel more tired during menopause, but that doesn't mean exercise is off the table. Instead, it's about tuning in to your body's rhythms and adjusting accordingly. If hitting the gym seems too daunting today, don't sweat it—literally. Perhaps a gentle yoga session or a brisk walk is more manageable, and that's okay. Listening to your body is the first step in crafting a routine that's as flexible as you need it to be.

Cardiovascular exercise remains a cornerstone of wellness, particularly in guarding against heart disease, which becomes more of a risk factor for women post-menopause. But consider the power of variety. If you're used to pounding the pavement, why not take a swim instead? It's gentle on the joints and can be incredibly soothing, making it a fantastic option for those days when you need a kinder approach to your body. Mixing up your cardio also keeps things fresh, helping you to stay engaged and less likely to skip a workout.

When it comes to building strength, weights can be your friends, but always start light and increase gradually. Muscle mass declines with age, which can impact everything from metabolism to bone density.

Weight training can help offset these changes, and it doesn't have to mean lifting heavy barbells. Bodyweight exercises, resistance bands, and light dumbbells can all be part of your strength-building toolkit. Remember, the goal is to empower, not overwhelm.

Balance and flexibility are two aspects we might overlook, yet they're critical during menopause. Incorporating postures and stretches that engage your core and improve your agility can help prevent falls and keep you limber. Simple balance exercises—like standing on one foot while brushing your teeth—can be seamlessly integrated into everyday life. And as for stretching, dedicating time to elongate and relieve your muscles can be a soothing ritual that also has practical benefits for mobility.

It's equally important to consider your schedule. Not everyone is an early bird, and plunging into a high-intensity workout first thing might not jive with your circadian rhythms. Instead, find a time when you feel most energetic—be it mid-morning or after work—and make that your regular workout slot. Being in tune with your body's clock can significantly impact the quality and consistency of your exercise routine.

Mind-body activities like Pilates, tai chi, and qi gong are great for engaging both your physical and mental faculties. These practices promote mindfulness, which can help battle menopausal symptoms like mood swings and anxiety. Plus, they're often low impact, making them sustainable for the long haul.

Don't mistake gentle for ineffective; often, lower-impact exercises can be profoundly transformative. Swimming, cycling, and even dancing can provide a cardiovascular workout that's friendly to your joints and uplifting for your spirits. Keeping the fun in your physical activity can be the motivation you need to keep moving, even on the tougher days.

When muscle soreness kicks in or a hot flash hits mid-session, remember that recovery and adjustments are vital. Take a day off if necessary, indulge in a long soak, or employ recovery tools like foam rollers. Your regimen isn't set in stone; it's meant to evolve with you, offering leeway for life's unpredictabilities, especially now.

Hydration is another non-negotiable. With sweat loss during exercise, it's imperative to drink plenty of water before, during, and after your workouts. Staying hydrated can help manage some menopausal symptoms and maintain your performance during exercise.

Finally, don't shy away from seeking guidance. A fitness trainer who understands the nuances of menopausal health can be an invaluable resource. They can help you craft and refine an exercise plan that takes into account your hormonal fluctuations, energy levels, and personal fitness goals.

Remember, your workout regimen is not just about maintaining your physical health; it's also instrumental in navigating the mental challenges of menopause. Regular physical activity can improve mood, enhance self-esteem, and provide a sense of accomplishment. These psychological wins are just as important as the physical gains.

Patience is paramount. Some days you'll feel strong and unstoppable; on others, it may feel like you're moving through molasses. Resist the urge to be critical and instead celebrate every small victory. Your body's response to exercise during menopause may be different from what it once was, but it's all part of the transition. Embrace it with kindness and understanding.

As you tailor your workout regimen, bear in mind that consistency is key. Find a rhythm that works for you and stick with it, but always allow room for flexibility. Life is not linear, and neither is menopause. Your workout plan should reflect the ebbs and flows of your journey, supporting you every step of the way.

Last but not least, keep your eye on the horizon. Fitness is not just about today's workout; it's about cultivating a sustainable lifestyle that will support you into post-menopause and beyond. By personalizing your fitness routine now, you're making an investment in your future self—one that will pay dividends in your physical endurance, mental resilience, and overall wellbeing.

So take a moment to connect with your body, assess your needs, and start building that perfect-fit workout regimen. The transition through menopause isn't just a phase; it's an opportunity to redefine and rediscover the strength and vitality within you. Embrace this chance to tailor your fitness to your life's new rhythm, and you'll emerge more robust and more grounded than ever before.

Chapter 9:
Cultivating Social Connections

In the rich tapestry of menopause management, the threads of social connections hold a special significance. As we wave goodbye to earlier chapters on diet and exercise, we nestle into the comforting embrace of relationships. The ebb and flow of hormones might tempt us to withdraw into solitude, but it's the power of community that often lights our way. Connections aren't just niceties; they're necessities, serving as both anchor and sail through menopausal seas. Sure, building bridges takes effort—reaching out, nurturing ties, and sometimes forging new paths. But let's remember, even if the thought of socializing feels as appealing as a hot flash in July, these connections form the lifeline to our well-being. As you read on, you'll absorb the hows and whys of establishing a support network that resonates with who you are and who you're blossoming into. It's about crafting bonds as unique as you are—authentic, strong, and unwavering in the face of change.

The Role of Social Support

As you navigate the complexities of menopause, the power of a strong social network becomes abundantly clear. It's about having those heartfelt conversations with friends, the ones where you laugh until your sides ache, or roll your eyes over the latest hot flash debacle, and it's also about the bonds you create with others who understand the turbulence of this season. These connections don't just brighten your day—they're lifelines, anchoring you to a community that nurtures your emotional well-being. Leaning on loved ones, joining support groups, or simply sharing stories over coffee can significantly reduce feelings of isolation and stress, allowing you to face the mental health challenges of menopause with a reinforced sense of solidarity. Remember, social support isn't a luxury; it's a crucial element in maintaining your mental equilibrium, providing both a mirror to reflect your experiences and a window to new approaches and perspectives. Embrace the camaraderie, let your guard down, and relish the embrace of those who've got your back—because together, you're unstoppable.

Creating and Maintaining Healthy Relationships

As we navigate the menopausal transition, the significance of healthy relationships cannot be overstated. These bonds can be a haven from the storm, offering support, understanding, and love as your body and mind undergo profound changes. However, maintaining relationships during this time can also present unique challenges. Let's dive into creating and caring for these vital connections, and learn how they can not only survive but thrive during menopause.

First, communication is key. It's crucial to articulate your needs and experiences during menopause. This isn't the time for subtleties. Be clear with your partner, family, and friends about what you're going through. Whether it's a need for quiet time or a shoulder to cry on, letting your loved ones know what you require helps them to be there for you in the most effective ways.

Furthermore, it's important to cultivate patience, both with yourself and others. Hormonal fluctuations can trigger irritability and mood swings, potentially leading to misunderstandings. Remember, those close to you might not fully comprehend the breadth of menopausal symptoms. Patience fosters a more empathetic environment where everyone is more inclined to work through conflicts with compassion.

Don't underestimate the power of empathy. Try to see situations from the perspective of your loved ones. They may feel helpless, watching you struggle and not knowing how to assist. Balance is key - while it's essential to advocate for your needs, also be open to their feelings and challenges.

Quality time together is vital. Engage in activities that both you and your loved ones enjoy. This can be as simple as a walk in the park, a movie night, or a shared hobby. Not only do these shared experiences bring joy, but they also reinforce the connection and provide a distraction from the rigors of menopause.

Remember to set boundaries. At times, you'll need space to process what you're going through, and that's okay. Make it clear that boundaries aren't barriers. They're integral to self-care and can make the time you do spend together even more meaningful.

Empower your loved ones with knowledge. Share resources about menopause with them. This isn't about them reading every book or article on the topic, but by understanding the basics, they can be more empathetic and proactive in supporting you.

Additionally, forge new social connections, particularly with those who empathize with your journey. Support groups, both in person and online, can provide a sense of camaraderie and mutual understanding. Connecting with peers who are going through similar experiences can be immensely grounding and reassuring.

Re-evaluate and adjust expectations. What worked in a relationship before menopause may need tweaking now. Recognize that change is part of life's natural rhythm and adapting can lead to even stronger relationships.

Acknowledge that sexuality may change during menopause, and approach this with openness and honesty. Intimacy can still be rich and fulfilling but may require new approaches or understanding from your partner. Be ready to explore and communicate to find a common ground that satisfies you both.

It's also a time to practice gratitude. Showing appreciation for the support you have can fortify relationships. Gratitude can effortlessly make your loved ones feel valued and motivate them to continue being supportive.

Stay mindful of your friendships. While family and partners are important, do not neglect your friends. Friendships provide variety and richness to your social life, offering different perspectives and support networks that can be just as valuable as familial or romantic relationships.

Seek out joy. Shared laughter can be a balm for the stress that menopause may bring into relationships. Look for the light-hearted moments and let them bring you closer together with those you care about.

Tackle challenges together. Viewing the menopausal transition as a team effort with your partner or loved ones can enhance solidarity. Working together to find solutions to the hurdles you face will build a stronger foundation for your relationships.

Remember to care for yourself too. You can't pour from an empty cup. Self-care is a crucial element that enables you to be present and engaged in your relationships. Prioritizing your well-being, through things like exercise, proper nutrition, and enough rest, equips you to be a more active and fulfilled participant in your relationships.

In conclusion, menopause is not a journey to walk alone. It offers an opportunity to deepen ties, learn new ways of relating, and rediscover the importance of community and connection. Healthy relationships during this stage of life require nurturing, compassion, and commitment, but the rewards are rich and immense. These relationships can provide a tapestry of support that not only sustains but strengthens you through menopause and beyond.

Chapter 10:
Cognitive Health and Menopause

As we close the page on nurturing the social garden of our lives, let's dive into the vibrant world of cognitive health during menopause. It's no secret that this transitional period can play a mischievous game with our minds, but it's not all doom and gloom. Imagine your brain as a muscle that craves its own kind of workout. Keeping your wits as sharp as a tack and your memory as sticky as a post-it note requires some dedicated mental gymnastics. We'll explore how to flex those neurons with mental exercises and brain training that not only enhance cognition but also inject a fun dose of 'brainplay' into your daily routine. Envision tackling puzzles, embracing new learning, and turning everyday tasks into brain-boosting challenges. It's about transforming the fear of cognitive decline into an actionable and uplifting journey of mental empowerment. Bring your curiosity, a zest for experimentation, and get ready to supercharge that brainpower!

Keeping Your Mind Sharp

As we continue to navigate the complexities of menopause, let's pivot our focus towards the vibrant realm of cognitive health. It's no secret that maintaining mental acuity can be a bit more challenging during this transition. Still, it's a game where strategy counts, and you've got the power to stay ahead. Picture your brain as a muscle that craves a good workout. Engaging in activities that require dexterity, such as puzzles, learning a new language, or even a musical instrument, can act as your mental gym. But, it's not just about intellectual gymnastics; social interaction, laughter, and embracing novel experiences all serve to kindle the synapses. Think of it as nurturing a garden in your mind

– it's about planting the seeds of curiosity and watering them with a mixture of wonder and discipline. Tend to it, and you'll reap the harvest of a sharper, more engaged intellect – a beacon guiding you through the foggy moments menopause might bring.

Mental Exercises and Brain Training Alright, stepping into the realm of cognitive health, it's crucial to engage the right strategies to support your brain - a bit like choosing the right pair of shoes for a run. You're traversing through a unique season of life, and your mental faculties need all the love and training they can get. Here, you're going to get a grip on exercises and activities that can flex those brain muscles, keeping your mind as fit as your body.

Mental fog might seem like an inevitable guest during menopause, but with the right exercises, you can show it the door. Let's talk about a workout, not for your physical self, but for the vibrant brain you carry. This is about building a brain gym - filled with puzzles, games, and new learning challenges that remind your neurons how to dance with agility and grace.

Let's highlight a favorite – the crossword puzzle. It's not just a lazy Sunday pastime; it's a powerful tool to fend off the cobwebs from your cognitive corridors. Crosswords challenge your recall, introduce you to new words, and force you to think in divergent ways. A perfect tool for you, as you transition through menopause, to keep the linguistic parts of your brain as sharp as a tack.

And how about learning a new language? There's a kind of magic that happens when you immerse yourself in learning Spanish, French, or even sign language. It's a fantastic way to enhance cognitive function, increase neural connections, and, as they say, a bilingual brain ages slower than a monolingual one. What better way to embrace this phase of life than with the excitement of a new form of communication?

Shifting gears - ever considered brain training apps? Yes, they're a thing. These apps are specifically designed to provide a series of exercises that improve memory, attention, and problem-solving skills. They're built on the science of neuroplasticity, which suggests that our brains can reorganize and form new connections, regardless of age. So, take advantage of technology and let your fingers guide you to a sharper mind.

Don't underestimate the simplicity of jigsaw puzzles either. They are both meditative and mental. As you sift through a sea of pieces, your brain is working on sorting, strategizing, and problem-solving. A jigsaw puzzle represents the messy beauty of life, which you can patiently piece together, one day at a time – a metaphor and a mental workout rolled into one.

Now let's focus on strategy games like chess or bridge – such cerebral pastimes! They demand your foresight, strategy, and memory. Engaging in these regularly not only passes the time but often leaves you with a sharper, more strategic mind. You'll find yourself better equipped to handle life's checkmates with poise.

The act of writing itself should not be overlooked. Whether it's journaling, poetry, or storytelling, writing nurtures creative thought and problem-solving. It's like a personal trainer coaxing your brain to build stronger neural pathways while you delve into self-expression. In these pivotal times, let yourself spill out onto pages; who knows what revelations about yourself are waiting to be penned?

Mathematics might have been a dreaded word in school, but guess what? It's cool again. Tackle Sudoku or engage in online math games. They force your brain to follow complex patterns, deeply engaging the logical parts of the mind. Each number puzzle solved is a small victory for your cognitive muscle.

They say you can't teach an old dog new tricks, but that's been proven wrong time and again. Take up a new hobby that requires fine motor skills, such as knitting, drawing, or playing a musical instrument. These hobbies not only produce beautiful results but also keep your brain engaged in learning and coordination, essential for maintaining cognitive health.

Remember, the brain thrives on variety. Rotate these exercises, mix them up, keep your brain guessing. It's the equivalent of cross-training; by challenging your mind in various ways, you're bolstering your mental resilience. You aren't just going through menopause, you're growing through it, and your brain's development is a testament to that progress.

Lastly, join a group or class. Whether it's a book club, an art class, or a chess club, the social interaction coupled with mental stimulation is an unbeatable combo. Socializing encourages active listening, empathy, and exchanging ideas - all of which enrich your cognitive processes and contribute to better emotional well-being during this significant transition.

Indeed, as you focus on mental exercises and brain training, you're laying the groundwork for a sharper, more engaged mind, prepared to embrace the nuances of menopause. Remember, it's not just about staying busy; it's about staying vibrant, relevant, and aware. Your cognitive health is an investment, and the dividends are profound.

Wrap up each day with a little reflection on how the mind exercises have impacted your day. Tracing the benefits reinforces the habit and deepens the appreciation for this stretch of life. Keep a log if you'd like, and watch as over time, the fog lifts, and clarity returns, ensuring that as you move through your menopausal journey, you're as mentally vibrant as you've ever been.

Now, with your arsenal of mental strategies, let's proceed to understand how you can complement these efforts with holistic therapies and alternative medicine. It's about supporting your brain and your emotional state from all fronts to navigate the menopausal voyage with grace and vigor.

Chapter 11:
Holistic Therapies and Alternative Medicine

ransitioning smoothly from the sharp tools of cognitive fortification presented previously, Chapter 11 opens up a garden of gentler options, where the petals of holistic therapies and the roots of alternative medicine intertwine to support your mental oasis. In this haven, natural remedies are not mere wisps of folklore; they are becoming a staunch ally in the menopausal journey, brimming with potential to alleviate mental tremors. This chapter is your guide to understanding how therapies like acupuncture can tap into the body's meridians to encourage equilibrium, while herbal supplements whisper promises of balance to your hormonal symphony. As you explore these verdant trails, we'll unearth how these practices, steeped in tradition, are gaining modern validation and how they offer a complementary approach to your mental wellness toolkit without any hint of condescension. Every herb, every needle-point, is a thread in the rich tapestry of options you can weave into your personalized menopausal tapestry.

Exploring Natural Remedies

Navigating the rollercoaster of menopause, you might find yourself seeking sanctuary in natural remedies—those gentle whispers of the earth beckoning to alleviate your turbulent symptoms. Truly, nature's apothecary is rife with options, from the humblest chamomile tea, which can soothe your nerves, to the flash of brilliance that is the evening primrose oil, a beacon for those wrestling with mood swings. It's about weaving these gifts into the tapestry of your wellness routine, discovering how a splash of valerian root may usher in the restorative sleep that's eluded you, or how the adaptogenic wonders of ashwagandha could lend balance to your hormonally besieged body. Remember, it's not about finding a miracle cure—those are the stuff of fairy tales—but about fostering harmony within. And while science might not back every petal and leaf with a resounding endorsement, every woman's menopausal odyssey is her own. So, let intuition guide you as you explore, incorporating these natural allies with discernment and a touch of hope, always in concert with your healthcare provider's sage advice.

The Benefits of Acupuncture and Herbal Supplements As the narrative of menopause unfolds, let's explore the realm of alternative medicine, namely acupuncture and herbal supplements, and their potential to alleviate some of the mental health challenges you may face during the menopausal transition. Imagine harnessing the ancient wisdom of these practices to navigate these changes with grace and vitality.

Acupuncture, a cornerstone of traditional Chinese medicine, involves the insertion of very fine needles into specific points on the body. The philosophy behind this practice is to stimulate the body's own healing processes. Interesting to note, acupuncture has been making waves in the West for its ability to help manage various menopausal symptoms, including those pesky mood swings and anxiety spells.

The experience of acupuncture is as unique as the individual receiving it. Some women report feeling energized after a session, while others bask in a calming afterglow. What's consistent, though, is the aim—balancing the body's energy flow, or 'Qi,' to promote mental and physical well-being. For many, the idea of balancing this flow fits perfectly with the quest for equilibrium during the hormonal variations of menopause.

Turning our gaze to the realm of herbal supplements, numerous natural remedies have been used over centuries to support health.

During menopause, these supplements can be particularly intriguing for their potential to ease symptoms without the need for pharmaceuticals. Herbs like black cohosh, red clover, and evening primrose oil are often the stars of the show, each bringing a blend of potentially symptom-alleviating effects.

Black cohosh, for example, has garnered attention for its ability to reduce hot flashes and improve mood. This botanical ally offers a natural approach to managing the ebbs and flows of menopausal symptoms, and for some, it might just be the missing puzzle piece to feeling more balanced.

With the change of life comes a shift in focus to what truly nourishes and supports our well-being. It's important to remember that herbs are potent, and while they're natural, they're not innocuous. Consulting a healthcare provider before diving into herbal supplementation is as imperative as it is sensible—it ensures that the path you're taking is as safe as it is healing.

Why consider these therapies? They're part of a broader palette of options available to you—a palette that's as diverse and rich as the experiences women have with menopause. Acupuncture and herbal supplements create opportunities to engage with your health in a proactive, personal way.

Indeed, studies have shown that acupuncture can help reduce stress and anxiety among menopausal women. The rationale behind this is believed to be linked to the practice's ability to modulate the stress-response axis. Essentially, it's like hitting a 'reset' button on your body's stress responses, giving you a chance to catch your breath and regroup.

Additionally, there's more to acupuncture than just needlework. It's often accompanied by an entire philosophy of care that includes lifestyle advice, dietary guidelines, and exercises like Tai Chi or Qigong. It's not just a treatment; it's a holistic approach to living well.

Speaking of living well, let's consider how herbal supplements can contribute to a more vibrant menopausal experience. Herbs like St. John's Wort have been highlighted for their potential to support mental health, particularly in alleviating depressive symptoms that can occasionally rear their head during menopause.

It's not just about symptom relief; it's about vitality. The holistic nature of these remedies encourages a broader view of health—one that encompasses the emotional, psychological, and physical dimensions of your being. Embracing these therapies can be part of a journey towards a deeper connection with yourself and a commitment to nurturing your overall wellness.

One cannot overlook the importance of quality and purity when it comes to selecting acupuncture practitioners and herbal supplements. It's crucial to seek certified professionals and high-quality, uncontaminated herbs. This due diligence is key to ensuring the benefits of these therapies are realized without unintended consequences.

A closing thought: embracing alternative therapies like acupuncture and herbal supplements during menopause is more than an act of self-care—it's a statement. It's declaring that you are the custodian of your well-being, open to exploring paths less trodden, and determined to navigate your transition with empowerment. It's recognizing that sometimes, the most profound healing comes from the most ancient of wisdoms.

While every woman's journey through menopause is different, acupuncture and herbal supplements offer a suite of options to consider for those looking to manage their mental health naturally and gently. With the right guidance and an openness to these age-old practices, you may just find the support you've been seeking as you navigate the ebb and flow of this pivotal stage of life.

In conclusion, as you continue to weave the fabric of your menopausal experience, remember that the choices you make—

including the decision to explore acupuncture and herbal supplements—have the power to influence your quality of life during this chapter. Your proactive steps today lay the groundwork for a more serene and fulfilling tomorrow. And isn't that what this transition is all about? A journey towards embracing a new rhythm, a new balance, and a renewed sense of self.

Chapter 12:
Hormone Therapy and Mental Health

As we sail through the waves of menopause, let's anchor at the port of hormone therapy and its ties to mental well-being. Hormone therapy can be a lighthouse amidst the fog, shedding light on the intricate dance between our hormones and our emotional landscape. What we're exploring in this chapter is the nuanced balance of risks and benefits that come with hormone therapy, always with an eye towards how it affects our mental health. Imagine a tailored ensemble, selected with care—such a personalized approach is key when considering hormone therapy for mental health during menopause. While blanket solutions don't fit everyone, understanding the common threads that bind hormones and mood can guide us in stitching together a plan that feels just right. It's about taking charge of your treatment, weighing options with a clear mind, and knowing that with the right information, you can make choices that help you stay afloat and even sail smoothly on your menopausal voyage.

Risks and Benefits

When considering hormone therapy for menopausal mental health, it's like standing at a crossroad with varied paths, each with its own set of milestones and hurdles. On the bright side, hormone therapy can be a game-changer for some, potentially easing those pesky mood swings, anxiety, and depressive episodes linked to plummeting estrogen levels. It's like turning on a light in a dim room; suddenly, things become clearer, and you may discover an uptick in your well-being. But don't be swayed without weighing the flip side—the risks. Yes, there can be side effects, and there's a delicate balance to maintain. We're talking about the nitty-gritty stuff like an increased risk of certain diseases. It's crucial to sync up with your healthcare provider to tailor a plan that's music to your body's unique rhythm, allowing you to savor the crescendo of benefits while sidestepping potential pitfalls. Remember, your menopausal journey should be harmonious with your health tune, empowering you to embrace every note of this life's symphony.

Personalized Treatment Plans When it comes to navigating the sometimes choppy waters of menopause, a one-size-fits-all approach is as effective as a screen door on a submarine. Personalization is the name of the game for hormone therapy and mental health management during this transformative time. And it's a game where you're in control, equipped with a map shaped by your unique circumstances. It is a journey of discovery, where the destination is your well-being.

Consider the rich tapestry of your life. Every woman experiences menopause differently, impacted by her own history, body chemistry, and lifestyle. This diversity is precisely why your treatment plan should be as unique as you are. Because when it comes to hormone therapy and mental health during menopause, what works for your best friend, sister, or neighbor may not be the best for you. Each treatment plan should be tailored with an understanding that you are unique, and so are your needs.

To start crafting your personalized treatment plan, consider starting with a detailed conversation with your healthcare provider. They can assess your symptoms, medical history, and preferences to help guide you towards therapy options that align with your goals. You might discuss family history, as it can provide insight into any potential genetic predispositions that could influence your treatment. It's integral to view this dialogue as a partnership, where your voice and comfort are central to the decision-making.

Personalized treatment plans may involve hormone therapy, but this is not an inevitable path for every woman. Hormone therapy can be incredibly effective for some, while others may experience better results with alternative approaches to manage their symptoms. It's important to weigh the risks and benefits carefully, considering factors such as current health, risk factors for diseases, and how menopausal symptoms impact your quality of life.

No two women will have the same risk profile, and thus, their hormone therapy regimens, if chosen, should reflect that individualized risk. For example, a woman with a personal or family history of breast cancer may opt for a different approach than a woman without such a history. An array of hormone therapies is available, from systemic therapies that affect the whole body to localized treatments that focus on specific symptoms, like vaginal dryness.

Even if you decide to incorporate hormone therapy into your plan, it's essential to view it as part of a broader holistic strategy. Mental health, so crucial during the menopausal transition, also benefits from a multidimensional approach. Therapy, support groups, stress management techniques, and other complementary practices can play a significant role in your mental and emotional well-being. It's important to create a mosaic of practices that work in harmony to support your health.

Monitoring and evaluating your treatment plan is an ongoing process. Adjustments can be necessary as your body responds or as your symptoms change. Keeping an open dialogue with your healthcare professional, and maintaining an awareness of your body's signals, allows for tweaking the plan to ensure it remains effective and suitable for you over time.

Your lifestyle choices are also an integral part of your personalized treatment plan. Nutrition, exercise, and sleep are pillars of general health that become even more important during menopause. We know that certain foods can influence hormone levels and mood, just as specific types of exercise can alleviate stress and support hormone balance. And let's not forget the importance of sleep, intimately connected with both mental and physical health.

When you're well-rested, nourished with brain-boosting foods, and engaged in physical activity that clears the fog and lifts your spirit, you've created a solid foundation. From this place, hormone therapy, if needed, can work more effectively, and any mental health strategies will be more potent because they're supported by a thriving body.

Let's not overlook the power of social connections in your treatment plan. The kind of support that friends, family, and support groups offer can't be bottled. Yet it's medicinal in its own right. Surrounding yourself with a community that understands and supports your journey can provide emotional sustenance that no medication can mirror.

In addition to discussions with your healthcare provider and personal research, tracking your symptoms can be invaluable in crafting and adjusting your treatment plan. By noting patterns in your mood, energy levels, and physical symptoms, you can work collaboratively to tailor your therapy extremely precisely, sometimes making small changes that result in significant improvements.

Remember, your treatment plan is dynamic, just like you. It's intended to evolve as you move through the different stages of menopause. Certain therapies or strategies may be more appropriate at one stage than another. It's a testament to the ongoing nature of self-care and self-discovery during menopause. This isn't a time for static solutions but for flexibility and responsiveness to your changing needs.

Making informed choices about your treatment plan can empower you. It can summon a sense of control in a phase of life often characterized by change. When you understand the why behind each aspect of your plan, it's easier to commit to and advocate for what you need. This is an opportunity to embrace your health journey with knowledge and confidence, knowing that your plan is tailor-made just for you.

In summary, your personalized treatment plan for hormone therapy and mental health during menopause isn't just a product of clinical recommendations. It's a living document, informed by your experiences, needs, preferences, and lifestyle. It's a pact between you and your health care provider, crafted to ensure your journey through menopause is as smooth and positive an experience as possible.

When you invest the time to develop a plan that aligns with who you are, you're committing to yourself, your mental health, and your overall well-being. And that's a commitment worth making. It's an opportunity to welcome change with courage, creativity, and a personalized roadmap to guide you through. Embrace your unique path to well-being – it's designed by you, for you, and it's as individual as your journey through menopause itself.

Chapter 13:
Self-Care Strategies

On this leg of the menopause journey, it's essential to remember that self-care isn't selfish; it's a non-negotiable for your well-being. Navigating menopause's choppy waters calls for a treasure map to self-care that's as unique as you are. Imagine weaving threads of joy into the fabric of daily life—maybe it's a morning ritual of sun salutations as the dawn whispers hello, or an evening gratitude journal that hugs you with the day's gifts. Self-compassion is your anchor, reminding you that it's okay to falter; it's a chance to wrap yourself in kindness and bounce back with grace. Let's not forget that laughter is a wellness tool, bubbling up joy right into your soul—it's like internal jogging for your mood. Crafting a self-care routine sows seeds for a flourishing garden within, where self-compassion blooms with the understanding that you're doing the best you can. And that's more than enough.

Developing a Self-Care Routine

As you journey through menopause, weaving a self-care routine into the fabric of your daily life can be a game-changer for your mental well-being. It's about carving out moments for yourself, celebrating small victories, and tuning in to your body's needs. Start simple: integrate activities that make you feel alive, whether it's sipping herbal tea while journaling or taking brisk walks in nature's embrace. Listen, your body's weathering a storm of hormonal shifts, and it's vital to create an oasis of calm amidst the whirlwind. Cultivate habits that nourish your soul and ground your mind—yoga might just become your newfound confidante. Remember, it's okay to start small and let your routine blossom organically; self-care isn't one-size-fits-all, it's about crafting a tapestry of practices that resonate with you. Your self-care routine is your personal haven; protect it fiercely, while also allowing it the flexibility to evolve with you through this transformative time.

The Importance of Self-Compassion as we navigate the complexities of menopause can't be overstated. You've been learning about the hormonal roller coaster, the nuances of mental health during this transition, and various coping mechanisms. Yet, in this sea of strategies and suggestions, there's a quiet buoy that often goes unnoticed: the role of self-compassion. Interestingly, as women, we're often taught to care for others, but taking a moment to extend that same kindness to ourselves can be a game-changer, particularly in the throes of menopause.

When we speak of self-compassion, we're digging into something more profound than self-care routines or stress relief tactics. We're examining the way we talk to ourselves during those absolutely human moments of struggle or self-doubt. Let's face it, hot flashes disrupting a night's sleep or a sudden wave of anxiety in the middle of a meeting isn't just uncomfortable; it's frustrating. But the way we respond to these challenges internally is critical.

Self-compassion is about acknowledging that these experiences are tough without falling into the trap of self-criticism. It's recognizing that menopause is a natural part of life—a shared experience among many women—and offers an opportunity for self-kindness. We can't control the tides of change, but we can certainly shift how we ride them, and doing so with compassion makes the journey more bearable.

Research consistently shows that individuals who practice self-compassion tend to have lower levels of stress and anxiety. Why? Because self-compassion helps to buffer the blow of difficult experiences, allowing for a soothing presence within. During menopause, when emotions and reactions can feel amplified, having this inner ally is precious.

Embracing self-compassion also fosters resilience. When faced with the various symptoms of menopause, from mood swings to memory fog, blaming ourselves for perceived inadequacies only adds to the stress. Instead, offering ourselves understanding and patience can help us to bounce back from setbacks more swiftly and effectively.

Interestingly, self-compassion can even play a role in physical health, with some studies suggesting that it can lead to better health habits and lower levels of inflammation. This is particularly important for menopausal women, given the increased risk of certain health issues during this time. Caring for our bodies starts with how we treat ourselves on the inside.

The key to self-compassion lies in treating ourselves as we would a good friend. If a friend were going through menopause, would we critique her for feeling overwhelmed or struggling with memory issues? Or would we offer words of encouragement and support? Finding ways to internalize this same sympathetic dialogue is transformative.

There's also a component of self-compassion that deals with mindfulness—being present with our feelings rather than avoiding or over-identifying with them. During menopause, you might feel a whirlwind of emotions. It's all too easy to either push them away or get swept up in them. Recognizing emotions as passing states that we don't have to judge or get lost in, brings a sense of peace.

And let's talk about those critical inner voices that tend to rear their heads during vulnerable times. Self-compassion asks us to silence those voices of self-doubt or harsh self-judgment. It's not about pretending everything is fine when it's not; it's about acknowledging the struggle while also affirming that it's okay to be imperfect. It's about allowing room for growth and learning without the harshness of self-reprimand.

In this time of change, acknowledging our strengths is also a part of self-compassion. Menopause doesn't negate the many incredible qualities you've nurtured over the years; it presents an opportunity to appreciate them even more. Perhaps you're a wonderful listener, a creative problem-solver, or someone who brings laughter to difficult situations. Celebrating these traits is just as important as being gentle with ourselves in moments of difficulty.

Implementing self-compassion into your life during menopause also means setting realistic expectations. Unrealistic goals or standards can lead to feelings of failure and self-criticism. It's crucial to understand that this period may come with limitations, and that's perfectly okay. Adjusting our objectives to reflect the current state of our body and mind is an act of kindness toward ourselves.

It's also immensely helpful to have compassionate role models—other women going through menopause who exude self-love and understanding. Their perspective can be both inspiring and relieving. It serves as a reminder that you're not alone, and that there are healthy, compassionate ways to handle this transition.

Lastly, self-compassion isn't a solo act. It includes reaching out for support when needed, whether that's talking to a trusted friend, joining a support group, or seeking professional guidance. It's recognizing when the burden feels too heavy and understanding that it's a sign of strength, not weakness, to ask for help.

In sum, self-compassion is a versatile and invaluable tool. It softens the edges of menopausal challenges and nourishes our emotional well-being. By integrating self-compassion into our lives, we're not just surviving menopause; we're thriving in it, with grace and love for ourselves as constant companions. This is as much a mental health strategy as any exercise or diet—perhaps even more so, because it starts within.

As we continue exploring ways to support your journey through menopause, let's not underestimate the transformative power of self-compassion. It's mighty yet gentle, and it has the potential to bring light into the more trying moments of your transition. Embrace it, practice it, and watch how it changes your menopausal experience for the better.

Transitioning Into Post-Menopause

As we turn the page from the myriad of changes encountered in the menopause journey, we embark on the steady state of post-menopause. Think of this phase as an opportunity to redefine your well-being, with a deeper understanding of your body's rhythms and needs. It's time to celebrate the resilience you've demonstrated and focus on the vibrant life that awaits. This stage brings with it a sense of stability, freed from the ebb and flow of hormonal fluctuations. With that stability comes a chance to realign your health priorities, ensuring that the lifestyle choices you make support your mental and physical health for the long term. You might notice that some symptoms linger or evolve, signaling that your relationship with your body is ever-changing and requires ongoing nurturing. Embracing these changes with a spirit of adaptability and optimism isn't just a feel-good mantra—it's a practical approach to thriving during post-menopause. So, as you plant your feet firmly in this new territory, let the steadiness of your internal landscape guide you towards fulfilling, healthful days filled with growth, joy, and the power that comes from an unwavering sense of self.

Preparing for the Next Phase

As we've pieced together the menopausal puzzle from psychological impacts to lifestyle adaptations, it's crucial to harness this knowledge for the road ahead. Post-menopause isn't merely an end to symptoms, but a vibrant stage where your well-being takes center stage. Imagine stepping forward with a wealth of strategies—from balancing nutrition to mindfulness practices that keep stress in check. Now, let's channel that wisdom into preparing for post-menopause. Over time, you've become adept at identifying mood shifts and adopting self-care rituals; it's time to lean into that resilience. Cultivate an environment that fosters cognitive sharpness and emotional vibrancy. We're talking about fine-tuning your regimen to navigate this transition smoothly, ensuring your mind and body are in sync. Keep in mind: this isn't just about dodging discomfort; it's about stepping into a life phase ripe with potential, armed with powerful tools and an indomitable spirit. Post-menopause can be your most empowering era yet, with your mental fortitude as the pinnacle of your journey.

Embracing Change and New Beginnings can be likened to drawing back the curtains to let in the sunlight after a restful night's sleep, even one that might've been interrupted a few times. Welcome to a section where we'll tie together the threads of transition and renewal, guiding you into a space where menopause isn't an ending but rather a passage to new adventures.

Imagine for a moment you're on a soft sandy beach. Each grain of sand represents a moment in your life, and you're keenly aware that some have slipped between your fingers as the waves of menopausal transition lap at your feet. But it's morning now, the tide is going out, and it leaves behind untrodden sand—a canvas for new experiences and opportunities.

Menopause marks a significant shift in a woman's life and it's not just a biological one. It's a time that often challenges one's identity, long-held beliefs about femininity, and can unearth anxieties about aging. But within this maelstrom of change, there's a powerful undercurrent that can propel you towards growth and discovery.

As the physical symptoms of menopause begin to settle, and you develop a newfound familiarity with this uncharted territory, there's a sense of empowerment that comes from having navigated those often turbulent waters. The key is to harness that fortitude and channel it into accepting change not just as an inevitable part of life, but as an invitation for new beginnings.

Discovering Fresh Passions and Priorities

With a transition like menopause, it's natural to reassess what truly matters to you. Perhaps you've dedicated years to nurturing others and now it's time to refocus some of that energy inward. What sparks joy in your life now? What goals have you set aside that are waiting to be dusted off? This period is ripe for exploration—a time to rekindle old passions or discover new ones.

Shifting Your Self-Perception

Change is often as much about perception as it is about physical reality. How you view yourself during and after menopause can profoundly affect your experience of it. You might be leaving behind the reproductive aspect of your womanhood, but you're stepping into a phase where wisdom, experience, and confidence can take the lead. Rebrand this time in your life as an era of new potential rather than loss.

Leveraging Life Experience

By now, you've collected a treasure trove of life experiences, lessons learned from both triumphs and defeats. These are not just keepsakes to look back on fondly; they are tools and strategies you can apply as you embrace the future. Recognize the strength drawn from these experiences and use them to navigate this new phase.

Reinventing Relationships

As you evolve, so too will your relationships. Friendships might shift, and family dynamics could change. It's an ideal time to evaluate who lifts you up and whom you might need to let go. Capitalize on the potential to deepen existing bonds or forge new ones that align with who you are in this season of life.

The Role of Community

Menopause can feel isolating, but it doesn't need to be a solo journey. There's immense power in community—sharing stories, wisdom, and support. Look around for groups or forums that can connect you with others walking a similar path. There's comfort in shared experiences, and often laughter and camaraderie await in these gatherings of kindred spirits.

Redefining Wellness

How you take care of yourself may change with menopause. The same activities, habits, or diets that served you well before might not have the same effect now. It's time to redefine what wellness means for you. Perhaps it's more gentle yoga and less high-impact aerobics, or maybe it's exploring meditation for the first time. Whatever form it takes, let wellness be an ever-evolving concept that suits your current needs.

Celebrating Your Evolving Identity

Your identity isn't static—it shifts and grows with you, and menopause can be a powerful catalyst in that growth. Celebrate the wisdom and maturity that come with your years. Embrace the changes in your body and mind as symbols of all you've lived through. Your evolving identity can be a badge of honor worn with pride.

Learning New Skills and Hobbies

Consider menopause a perfect excuse to expand your horizons. Always wanted to learn to paint? Interested in gardening? It's never too late to pick up new skills or hobbies. Delight in the process of learning and appreciate how it can enrich your life and keep your mind sharp.

Financial Planning for the Future

As your personal and professional life might be shifting, so too should your financial planning. This fresh chapter is the perfect time to reassess financial goals and ensure they reflect your current and future aspirations. Look at your finances through the lens of possibility and security for this new stage.

Anticipating Post-Menopausal Health

Keeping an eye on what lies ahead health-wise can do wonders for your peace of mind and physical well-being. Now's a good time to understand how your health needs will change post-menopause and what you can do to stay ahead of the game. This proactive approach is both empowering and reassuring.

As you stand at the precipice of post-menopause, remember that the horizon is wide and filled with a myriad of possibilities. It's an expanse that calls for exploration, curiosity, and joy. Embrace change as a companion that whispers of new dawns, fresh hopes, and untold stories waiting to be lived.

While menopause may be a conclusion to a particular part of your life, it's the prologue to a fascinating new volume. Transform this time into an opportunity to ignite your creativity, invigorate your lifestyle, and inspire those around you. You've weathered the storm, now dance in the sunlight of new beginnings.

Chapter 15:
Building Your Menopausal Mental Wellness Plan

After exploring the various dimensions of menopausal changes, it's clear that while the journey is deeply personal, crafting a proactive approach for mental wellness is something we all can benefit from. It's about tuning into your body's signals, recognizing the subtle shifts, and honoring them with strategies that truly resonate with your needs. In this chapter, we're rolling up our sleeves to put together a mental wellness plan that isn't just a cookie-cutter solution—it's tailored to the ebb and flow of your unique menopausal experience. We'll dive into setting realistic goals that don't just sit on a to-do list but integrate seamlessly into your life. It's about creating a living document—your personalized blueprint—that evolves as you do, allowing for reflection, tracking progress, and making those small adjustments that can lead to significant leaps in your mental wellbeing. Whether it's integrating a few mood-boosting activities into your weekly routine or carving out the time for self-reflection, the aim is to construct a resilient mental framework that supports you through the ripples of menopause. Remember, this isn't about getting it perfect—it's about making space for growth, understanding, and kindness towards yourself as you navigate this pivotal chapter.

Setting Realistic Goals

Embarking on your mental wellness journey during menopause necessitates setting attainable objectives that steer your paths without overwhelming you. Imagine sculpting a personal masterpiece, where each deliberate chisel strike counts—it's about progress, not perfection. Start by establishing specific, measurable goals that align with your lifestyle and capabilities. Rather than aiming for a complete overhaul, consider incremental changes; think improvements in sleep quality, manageable stress-relief practices, or nourishment tweaks that boost cognitive function. Recognize this life phase's unique challenges and remember to celebrate every victory, no matter how petite. Your hormonal milieu may be in flux, but your aspirations should be grounded in kindness toward yourself and a strong belief in attainable growth. **Commit to your menopausal mental wellness** with reachable milestones that empower you, and watch as your well-being blossoms, transforming challenges into triumphs.

Tracking Progress and Adjusting As Needed

Having gracefully set foot into this sacred space of understanding and managing one's mental health during the menopausal transition, the journey now segues into nurturing a crucial element of our wellness crusade: tracking progress and the art of making necessary adjustments. Let's embark on carving pathways toward not just adapting but thriving in this chapter of life.

Embarking on a path toward improved mental health during menopause means acknowledging the fluidity of this experience. Just as the body's needs fluctuate, so do the desires and demands of the mind. This is where tracking progress shines – it's about having a clear picture of where you're at and where you're headed, akin to navigating a roadmap studded with your personal milestones and scenic routes of self-discovery.

Scrupulously documenting your feelings, symptoms, and overall wellbeing in a journal or digital tracker can offer illuminating insights. Charting the ebb and flow of your mood, the quality of sleep, or the vim brought by exercise demonstrates glimpses into the effectiveness of your coping strategies. It's a practice that encourages mindfulness while illuminating patterns the astute mind might miss.

How do you feel after a brisk walk or a hearty chat with a friend? Capture it. The key here is consistency. Regular check-ins serve as echoes of your experience, providing a space for reflection, and functioning as waypoints for further exploration and adjustment. Keep it simple and achievable – let's eschew elaborate schemes for simple, daily logs that speak your truth.

Embrace the trial-and-error nature of this process. There's no one-size-fits-all answer when it gets down to navigating menopause. If certain dietary changes aren't yielding the desired results, it's a cue to pivot or consult with a nutritionist. Tweak your self-care rituals, exercise routines, or mindful practices if they seem to falter in their magic. Change is your ally, not your foe.

It's also essential to recognize patterns. Maybe you'll notice that your mood tends to dip during certain times of the month or that stressful days at work lead to disrupted sleep. These revelations, while sometimes subtle, can greatly influence the course of action you take to adjust your mental wellness plan.

Digging a bit deeper, consider the impact of your social connections. Are they nourishing or draining you? Utilize your tracked insights to discern which relationships bolster your mental health and which may necessitate boundaries. Building and maintaining uplifting relationships is a dynamic process that benefits from regular check-ins and honest evaluations.

Measurement can also extend to tracking cognitive changes. Keeping your mind sharp might involve memory exercises, puzzles, or learning new skills. By measuring your cognitive activities and their frequency, you can assess what's working or where you may need to challenge yourself further to maintain mental acuity.

Let's not forget about the role of laughter, joy, and creativity in your mental health journey. These too deserve a spot in your progress tracker. Noting down activities that bring you happiness is just as critical as monitoring symptoms. After all, menopause – while challenging – is also a time ripe for rediscovery and joy.

Amongst these endeavors, be patient and gentle with yourself. Adjustments should be realistic, celebrating small victories rather than expecting dramatic leaps. It's the subtle shifts and gentle, sustained efforts that often lead to the most profound changes.

Sometimes you'll notice progress isn't linear. Setbacks happen. It's all a part of the great ebb and flow of life. Don't be disheartened when the waters become choppy; remember, the most skilled sailors aren't defined by smooth seas but by their ability to sail in all conditions. Accept the natural rhythm of your journey, knowing that with each recalibration, you gather more wisdom.

At times, it might be beneficial to share this journey with a healthcare provider or a therapist, especially if adjustments seem daunting or symptoms intensify. Collaboration can lead to innovative solutions and provide you the support needed to brave this transformative era.

As you move forward, keep an eye on long-term trends. The nuances of self-improvement often hide in overarching trajectories rather than in day-to-day flux. Over time, your diligent tracking will morph into an invaluable chronicle that reflects not just where you've been but illuminates where you're headed – toward a state of thriving wellness.

In the end, remember that tracking your progress isn't about perfection; it's about progression. It's about harnessing the power of self-awareness to fuel positive change and ensuring your menopausal mental wellness plan grows and breathes with you. Engage in this practice with an explorer's heart – open to learning, adapting, and navigating the beautiful landscape of menopause with grace and intention.

You're the cartographer of your own voyage. May tracking your progress and adjusting your sails as necessary lead you to tranquil waters and bright horizons. Each step you take is a testament to your courage and a stitch in the vibrant tapestry of your life. Onward with tenacity and hope, for this journey's narrative is yours to write.

The Confident Self Beyond Menopause

As we've journeyed together through the different facets of menopause, we've gathered an arsenal of wisdom, tools, and strategies to handle the mental health challenges that come with this transition. Now, we stand at a point where we can confidently say that menopause is not an endpoint, but a passage to a new phase of life where self-assurance and well-being are within reach. The culmination of this exploration brings us to the heart of what it means to live confidently beyond menopause.

Embracing your post-menopausal self is about more than just coping with symptoms; it's a holistic embrace of the change in your life's seasons. Just as we anticipate spring after the chill of winter, so too can we look forward to the new growth post-menopause brings. This period can be a time of unprecedented freedom, discovery, and inner strength, as we let go of old constraints and embrace new possibilities.

The key to forging this new identity lies in the heart of resilience. Resilience isn't just bouncing back; it's about bending and not breaking, adapting to change, and coming out stronger. It's about recognizing that the hormonal turbulence and the psychological upheaval have equipped you to deal with any storms that lie ahead with a calm and steady hand.

Menopause is often depicted as a loss, a decline, or even an unwelcome disruption to life as we know it. It's high time we flip the narrative and see it as a time of gaining—gaining wisdom, gaining time for ourselves, gaining new perspectives. Embrace your story with all its imperfections because it's in the embracing that we find acceptance and, ultimately, peace.

The journey to this point has likely given you a deeper understanding of your mental health and the crucial role self-care plays. No longer an afterthought, nurturing your well-being has hopefully become an integral part of your daily life. Prioritizing self-compassion and embracing practices that bolster your mental state can continue to serve as your compass, guiding you to calmer waters.

Remember all the strategies we've talked about for managing stress, nourishing your body, and engaging your mind? They're not just methods to get you through menopause; they're lifestyle adaptations to carry you through the rest of your life. Integrating mindfulness, exercise, nutrition, and cognitive exercises into your routine isn't just beneficial; it's transformative.

Post-menopausal life is ripe with opportunity for personal development. It's a testimony to your ability to overcome and a platform to inspire others entering this phase of life. Your confidence is a beacon, shining as proof of your journey through the menopausal transition and, most importantly, of your growth and triumph beyond it.

The social connections you've cultivated and maintained throughout menopause? They're the bedrock upon which your post-menopausal life will flourish. The support of friends, family, and other like-minded individuals will continue to be a source of strength and joy as you embark on new adventures with the confidence of your hard-won self-knowledge.

And let's not forget the therapeutic options, from holistic remedies to hormone therapy, that you've explored in these pages. These are tools at your disposal, choices to make based on personal preference and medical advice, and they serve to underscore your autonomy over your health and happiness.

Looking beyond to the horizon, setting realistic goals, and tracking your progress, opens up a world of fulfillment and self-actualization. As you adjust your sails for the post-menopausal journey, take pride in setting goals that reflect your values, your passions, and your newfound confidence.

Imbued with this mindset, the transition into post-menopause becomes not just manageable, but something to be approached with a sense of anticipation and excitement. Embracing change is not merely about reconciling with a new phase of life; it's an active process of shaping that life assertively and enthusiastically.

Your menopausal mental wellness plan doesn't end here; it evolves with you. The goals you set, the insight you've gained, and the strategies you've employed are parts of a growing, breathing blueprint for your well-being. It is adaptable, just like you, and designed to support your journey toward the best version of yourself.

With each chapter of this book, we've built up layers of understanding, compassion, and strategies for thriving. Now, as we close, these layers solidify into a foundation upon which you can stand tall and face the future with confidence. Your post-menopausal self is not just about surviving; it's about thriving, leading, and inspiring.

The confident self beyond menopause is a force to be reckoned with. She is not defined by the cessation of her menstrual cycle but by the depth of her experiences, the strength of her spirit, and the glow of her personal achievements. As you navigate beyond the menopausal transition, carry with you the certainty that this next stage can be as vibrant, impactful, and fulfilling as any other.

In closing, let's celebrate this new chapter. Each day is a canvas, and you hold the brush. Paint your days with the confidence of someone who has mastered the art of self-care, the grace of someone who knows herself deeply, and the excitement of someone ready to leave a unique mark on the world. The confident self beyond menopause is not just an idea – it is you: renewed, resilient, and radiant.

Appendix A: Appendix

As we come to the end of our exploration into menopause and mental health, you're likely feeling empowered with knowledge and ready to take on this transition with a renewed sense of confidence. But the journey doesn't end here. The Appendix is designed as a toolkit to help you further customize your personal wellness strategy as you navigate through menopause with grace and vigor.

A. Resources for Further Reading

Arm yourself with wisdom. Knowledge is not only power—it's also peace of mind. Delve deeper into the menopausal labyrinth with an array of books, articles, and websites dedicated to every facet of your transition. You will find that the more you know, the more you can anticipate and understand the nuances of your body and mind.

B. Relaxation Techniques

Breathe in calmness and exhale stress. In this section, you'll find a curation of relaxation techniques that you can infuse into your daily routine. From simple breathing exercises to more involved practices, these methods can help you maintain a serene mindset amid the waves of hormonal changes.

C. Self-Assessment Tools for Menopausal Symptoms

Listening to your body and tracking your symptoms is like drawing your own personal health map. The tools provided here will guide you in monitoring your signs and symptoms, helping you and your healthcare provider craft a plan that truly aligns with your individual experience.

Remember, each woman's journey through menopause is unique. Some days will feel like a breeze, while others may challenge your resolve. It's all about finding balance and tools that resonate with your life. Lean into this time of transformation, and let your instincts and the resources in this appendix guide you to a place of well-being. You've got this!

A. Resources for Further Reading

As you've journeyed through the chapters of this book, gaining insight and tools for navigating menopause and its related mental health challenges, you may find yourself yearning for more information. This section is dedicated to guiding you toward a wealth of resources that extend your knowledge and provide additional support as you continue on your path of personal growth and well-being.

One of the great things about our times is the abundance of information at our fingertips, and when it comes to menopause, there's no shortage of excellent reading material. For those looking to delve deeper into the scientific aspect of hormonal changes and their psychological impact, numerous books offer comprehensive insights. Start with titles that break down complex biological processes into understandable language, so you're not only gaining knowledge but also empowering yourself with information that makes sense to you.

Understanding the myths and facts about menopause is also critical. Seek out books that dispel common misconceptions and equip you with factual information. Misinformation can breed unnecessary fear or embarrassment, and by educating ourselves, we can counter those negative feelings with confidence and clarity.

Depression, anxiety, and mood swings can be a troublesome trio during the menopausal transition. It's vital to explore resources that provide strategies for managing these symptoms. Look for books coauthored by health professionals and psychologists that offer evidence-based methods for dealing with mental health challenges. They often include relatable anecdotes, making the guidance provided both practical and inspirational.

Positive thinking is more potent than you may realize, and several authors have tackled this subject with a blend of motivational narratives and scientific backing. Search for works that not only inspire you but also provide practical exercises for reframing your thoughts and expectations. An excellent resource should bridge the gap between understanding the power of positivity and actually applying it in your day-to-day life.

For those grappling with stress and anxiety, literature on mindfulness and relaxation techniques can be incredibly beneficial. Choose resources that offer step-by-step instructions on meditation or breathing exercises. A good book will help you develop a more intimate understanding of your body's responses to stress and how to soothe yourself in moments of tension.

Don't underestimate the importance of nurturing your emotional well-being. There's a range of texts that highlight the significance of emotional expression and building emotional resilience. Opt for those that provide empathetic guidance, encouraging you to face your emotions with courage and develop techniques to recover from setbacks more robustly.

Sleep is crucial, and sleep disruptions during menopause can be particularly vexing. Look for resources that discuss strategies for improving sleep quality and provide a deep dive into how hormonal changes can affect sleep patterns. Well-researched books can often present solutions that you may not have considered before.

There's a fascinating link between nutrition and cognitive health, and many authors have explored this connection. Find comprehensive guides that list brain-boosting foods and discuss the role of supplements for maintaining cognitive health. These resources can be invaluable in designing a diet that supports mental sharpness.

Exercise isn't just about keeping fit; it's about staying mentally clear as well. Dive into literature that elaborates on the mental benefits of physical activity and offers guidance on tailoring workouts to your unique stage in life. The right resource can motivate you to move your body in ways that feel good and benefit your mental wellness.

Social connections play a major role in our mental health. With profound changes happening during menopause, maintaining and creating healthy relationships can sometimes be challenging. Look for books that provide insights into the role of social support networks and practical tips for nurturing those connections.

Finally, as you look toward the future, gaining understanding in cognitive health during menopause can be empowering. Choose educational materials that highlight cognitive exercises, brain training, and keeping your mind sharp as you age. You'll find that these resources often mix science with motivational stories to inspire ongoing mental engagement.

It's also wise to consider exploring resources that discuss holistic therapies and alternative medicine. These can offer fresh perspectives on managing menopause symptoms. Select books that provide balanced views, ensuring that you have all the information needed to make informed decisions about your body and health.

Hormone therapy can be a significant aspect of the menopausal journey for many. Read up on the latest findings, risks, benefits, and personalized treatment plans through up-to-date and expertly researched material. Knowing your options, in the long run, is key to making choices that align with your values and health goals.

Self-care is a continuous theme throughout this book and looking to additional literature for deepening that practice is encouraged. Seek out resources that help in developing a comprehensive self-care routine, delve into the importance of self-compassion, and provide guidance on how to remain dedicated to these practices as life evolves.

Last but not least, building your post-menopause life can be an exciting adventure. Sources that focus on embracing change and finding new beginnings can serve as excellent companions as you transition into this next phase. Select books that resonate with this transformative period, offering both reflective insights and actionable advice.

Whether you're just beginning to explore the world of menopause or looking to expand your knowledge and coping strategies, there's a wealth of resources available. Take your time, find books and guides that speak to you, and remember that your journey is yours alone – and it's one worth navigating with all the support and knowledge you can gather.

B. Relaxation Techniques

Navigating the menopausal transition can be a puzzle of managing physical changes and the emotional whirlwind that accompanies them. Now, let's take a deep dive into a treasure trove of relaxation techniques that could be your guiding light during these transformative years. It's time to find that soothing calm amidst the storm—to empower you to grasp the reins of your mental health with grace and confidence.

Firstly, let's talk about the art of deep breathing. Yes, it's an art because it takes practice to truly harness its power. It's the simplest form of relaxation yet one of the most powerful. When you're feeling the heat rising—not just from hot flashes, but stress too—try this: find a comfortable seat, close your eyes, and inhale deeply through your nose, allowing your abdomen to expand fully. Hold this breath for a moment, then exhale slowly through your mouth. Repeat this cycle for a few minutes, and feel the tension begin to lift.

Visualization is another splendid tool. Picture yourself in a serene setting, perhaps a lush garden or a peaceful beach. With every in-breath, imagine drawing in calmness, and with each out-breath, envisage blowing away any unease. This mental escape can lower your stress levels and provide a healing mental break.

Progressive muscle relaxation is like giving your body a message to 'power down.' Start by tensing a group of muscles as you breathe in, hold for a few seconds, then release them as you breathe out. Move through each muscle group, from your toes to your forehead. It's a physical act with significant mental benefits, helping to diminish anxiety and improve sleep.

Guided imagery taps into the power of your mind to transport you to a place of tranquility. There are plenty of guided recordings available—each a verbal path leading you through landscapes of relaxation. They're especially useful when you're struggling to quiet a busy mind before sleep.

Yoga isn't just about striking a pose; it's a holistic practice that balances the body and mind. The gentle stretching, controlled breathing, and meditative elements of yoga can substantially reduce stress levels. Plus, it's adaptable for all fitness levels, making it an inclusive option for menopausal women seeking solace and strength.

Tai chi, often described as 'meditation in motion,' is another form of gentle exercise that can combat menopausal stress. Its flowing movements can help center your thoughts, improve your mood, and foster a sense of peace.

Autogenic training involves a series of self-statements about heaviness and warmth in different parts of your body. While saying these phrases, you're directing your body to enter a state of relaxation. This technique can help refocus your mind and alleviate symptoms of stress.

Mantra meditation involves the repetition of a calming word or phrase to prevent distracting thoughts. It's a beacon that guides your mind back to a state of rest whenever it starts to wander with worries or to-do lists.

Aromatherapy harnesses the soothing power of scent. Essential oils, from calming lavender to uplifting citrus, can significantly impact your mood. Add a few drops to a bath or diffuser, and let the fragrance carry you to a more tranquil mental space.

Journaling can be incredibly therapeutic. It's an outlet for the swirling thoughts and emotions that may arise during menopause. Pouring your heart onto the page can be cathartic, offering clarity and a greater sense of calm.

Listening to relaxing music sets the tone for a relaxed mindset. Whether it's classical melodies or the sounds of nature, allow the music to envelop you and replace your worries with harmonious peace.

Qigong, a practice closely related to Tai chi, is a system of coordinated body-posture, movement, breathing, and meditation used for health, spirituality, and martial arts training. Like Tai chi, it promotes inner peace and calm.

Finally, do not underestimate the power of laughter—it truly can be the best medicine. Whether you're sharing a chuckle with friends or enjoying your favorite comedy, laughter can reduce stress hormones and increase the feel-good chemicals in your brain.

Massage therapy is well-known for its ability to relieve physical tension, but it's just as effective for mental stress. If professional massages aren't an option, even a simple self-massage can work wonders for relaxation.

As you explore these relaxation techniques, remember that there's no one-size-fits-all solution. Menopause is a personal journey, and what works for one woman might not for another. It's all about finding the tools that resonate with you, bringing you back to a place of balance and rekindling the joy and peace within yourself. As you move through each day of your menopausal transition, keep these strategies in your back pocket and pull them out whenever you need a moment of reprieve. Your mental health is just as critical as your physical health, and nurturing it with these techniques will help ensure you flourish during menopause and beyond.

C. Self-Assessment Tools for Menopausal Symptoms

As we close one chapter and gently step into another, let's usher in the tools you need to assess and understand the landscape of your menopausal symptoms. Self-assessment tools aren't just questionnaires; they're keys that unlock a deeper understanding of your unique experiences. They help paint a more vivid picture of where you are on your menopausal journey and how it's impacting your mental and emotional well-being.

The beauty of these tools lies in their ability to quietly whisper the nuances of your body's changes when sometimes they feel like they're shouting. By taking inventory of your symptoms and their severity, you can recognize patterns, make informed decisions about your health, and communicate more effectively with healthcare providers.

Begin with a simple checklist. This isn't your ordinary grocery list—think of it as a contemplative composition of what you're experiencing. Hot flashes, night sweats, irregular periods, mood swings, and anxiety are all common markers for menopause. But remember, your checklist is personal. It might include symptoms not commonly discussed, like changes in memory or concentration, a sense of loss, or even newfound liberation.

Let's turn the spotlight on journaling. Not only does it serve as a cathartic release, but it's also a treasure trove of insight into your day-to-day experiences. Capture how you feel mentally, the quality of your sleep, dietary choices, and any episodes of stress or anxiety. Over time, your journal becomes a rich narrative of your menopausal transition, one that helps you and your healthcare team create a tailored approach to your well-being.

One of the more structured approaches involves symptom scales and questionnaires, many of which are validated by the medical community. The Menopause Rating Scale (MRS), for example, can provide a broad overview of your present situation. It's like having a conversation with yourself, one question at a time, about how menopause is influencing your life.

Another valuable resource is the Greene Climacteric Scale, which dives deeper into psychological symptoms. Remember, mental health is just as crucial as physical health during this transformative period. By pinpointing issues like anxiety and depression, such tools help in decoding the complex interplay of menopause and mental well-being.

Tracking apps are the modern woman's diary. With a tap and a swipe, you can monitor the frequency and intensity of symptoms. Many apps let you note additional factors such as diet, exercise, and sleep patterns. This digital log is exceptionally handy for spotting trends and emerging patterns in your menopause experience.

For those who prefer a more tech-savvy approach, wearable devices provide data on sleep quality, heart rate variability, and even predict hot flash occurrences based on body temperature. The gadgets are getting smarter, and so should we in utilizing technology to decode the language of our bodies.

Online questionnaires and calculators give a quantitative edge to the qualitative experience of menopause. By inputting symptoms and their frequency, these tools can offer immediate feedback, like an initial gauge of the severity of your symptoms or the effectiveness of current management strategies.

Factor in a symptom impact questionnaire to shed light on how menopausal changes are affecting your daily life. This goes beyond mere frequency; it assesses the ripple effect symptoms have on your work, social interactions, and inner peace.

Peer support forums are a treasure chest of shared knowledge and experiences. While not a traditional self-assessment tool, these forums can provide a sense of solidarity and unexpected insights as you read stories mirroring your own or discover symptoms you hadn't realized were connected to menopause.

Another avenue to explore is mood charts. Mood swings can be as unpredictable as a stormy sea. Charting your moods day by day, you'll begin to map out patterns. Maybe you'll notice that your mood dips correlate with certain sleep patterns or nutrition habits, giving you actionable information for lifestyle adjustments.

Tallying your symptoms can give rise to the bigger picture of your menopausal transition. It's a simple concept: you mark down symptom occurrences and their intensity, allowing you to visualize frequency and associations over time.

Remember to review these assessment tools regularly. Just as your life changes, so does your menopausal journey. Regular check-ins with your toolkit can indicate whether your management strategies are effective or if it's time to adapt and explore new avenues for relief.

Be mindful, as self-assessment tools aren't a substitute for professional medical advice. They're allies in your endeavor; tools meant to complement the guidance you receive from your healthcare team. And with their aid, you're better equipped to articulate your needs with precision and confidence.

As you weave these tools into the fabric of your daily life, they should invigorate you with empowerment. Knowing where you stand gives you the power to step forward in the direction you choose. So, grab that pen, tap that app, sync that device and let's map the rich, complex terrain of your menopausal experience with clarity and courage.

Equipped with self-awareness and these tools, the next chapter in your journey becomes less about what menopause is doing to you and more about what you're doing with menopause—managing, adapting, thriving. Just remember, this phase is your own unique story, and with these resources, it's one where you hold the pen firmly in hand, ready to script a tale of resilience, growth, and joy.

www.ingramcontent.com/pod-product-compliance
Lightning Source LLC
Chambersburg PA
CBHW030410290526
45785CB00004B/1959